TEENAGE
SEX:

WHAT SHOULD SCHOOLS TEACH CHILDREN?

Institute of Ideas
Expanding the Boundaries of Public Debate

TEENAGE SEX:

WHAT SHOULD SCHOOLS TEACH CHILDREN?

Institute of Ideas
Expanding the Boundaries of Public Debate

Ellie Lee and Tiffany Jenkins
David J. Landry
Simon Blake
Janine Jolly
Stuart Waiton
Peter Hitchens
Peter Tatchell

Hodder & Stoughton

A MEMBER OF THE HODDER HEADLINE GROUP

DEBATING MATTERS

Orders: please contact Bookpoint Ltd, 130 Milton Park, Abingdon, Oxon OX14
4SB. Telephone: (44) 01235 827720. Fax: (44) 01235 400454.
Lines are open from 9.00 - 6.00, Monday to Saturday, with a 24 hour message
answering service. Email address: orders@bookpoint.co.uk

British Library Cataloguing in Publication Data
A catalogue record for this title is available from
the British Library

ISBN 0 340 84834 0

First Published 2002
Impression number   10 9 8 7 6 5 4 3 2 1
Year   2007 2006 2005 2004 2003 2002

Typeset by Transet Limited, Coventry, England
Printed in Great Britain for Hodder & Stoughton Educational, a division of
Hodder Headline Plc, 338 Euston Road, London NW1 3BH by Cox & Wyman,
Reading Berks.

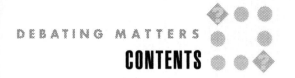

DEBATING MATTERS

CONTENTS

DEBATING MATTERS

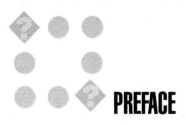

PREFACE

Since the summer of 2000 the Institute of Ideas (IOI) has organized a wide range of live debates, conferences and salons on issues of the day. The success of these events indicates a thirst for intelligent debate that goes beyond the headline or the sound-bite. The IOI was delighted to be approached by Hodder & Stoughton, with a proposal for a set of books modelled on this kind of debate. The *Debating Matters* series is the result and reflects the Institute's commitment to opening up discussions on issues which are often talked about in the public realm, but rarely interrogated outside academia, government committee or specialist milieu. Each book comprises a set of essays, which address one of four themes: law, science, society and the arts and media.

Our aim is to avoid approaching questions in too black and white a way. Instead, in each book, essayists will give voice to the various sides of the debate on contentious contemporary issues, in a readable style. Sometimes approaches will overlap, but from different perspectives and some contributors may not take a 'for or against' stance, but simply present the evidence dispassionately.

Debating Matters dwells on key issues that have emerged as concerns over the last few years, but which represent more than short-lived fads. For example, anxieties about the problem of 'designer babies', discussed in one book in this series, have risen over the past decade. But further scientific developments in reproductive technology, accompanied by a widespread cultural distrust of the implications of these developments, means the debate about 'designer babies' is set to continue. Similarly, preoccupations with the weather may hit the news at times of flooding or extreme weather conditions, but the underlying concern about global warming and the idea that man's intervention into nature is causing the world harm, addressed in another book in the *Debating Matters* series, is an enduring theme in contemporary culture.

At the heart of the series is the recognition that in today's culture, debate is too frequently sidelined. So-called political correctness has ruled out too many issues as inappropriate for debate. The oft noted 'dumbing down' of culture and education has taken its toll on intelligent and challenging public discussion. In the House of Commons, and in politics more generally, exchanges of views are downgraded in favour of consensus and arguments over matters of principle are a rarity. In our universities, current relativist orthodoxy celebrates all views as equal as though there are no arguments to win. Whatever the cause, many in academia bemoan the loss of the vibrant contestation and robust refutation of ideas in seminars, lecture halls and research papers. Trends in the media have led to more 'reality TV', than TV debates about real issues and newspapers favour the personal column rather than the extended polemical essay. All these trends and more have had a chilling effect on debate.

But for society in general, and for individuals within it, the need for a robust intellectual approach to major issues of our day is essential. The *Debating Matters* series is one contribution to encouraging contest about ideas, so vital if we are to understand the world and play a part in shaping its future. You may not agree with all the essays in the *Debating Matters* series and you may not find all your questions answered or all your intellectual curiosity sated, but we hope you will find the essays stimulating, thought provoking and a spur to carrying on the debate long after you have closed the book.

Claire Fox, Director, Institute of Ideas

NOTES ON THE CONTRIBUTORS

Simon Blake is Director of the Sex Education Forum. He is a member of the Independent Advisory Group for the Government's Teenage Pregnancy Strategy, an assessor for the National Healthy School Standard and a member of the National Sexual Health Strategy development group. Simon has written and contributed to a number of publications including *STRIDES: a practical guide to sex and relationships education with young men* (1998); *Moving Goalposts: setting a training agenda for sexual health work with boys and young men!* (2001); and *Just Say No! to Abstinence Education: A report of a sex education study tour to the US* (2001).

Peter Hitchens is a columnist for the *Mail on Sunday*, the author of *The Abolition of Britain* and *Monday Morning Blues* and is currently at work on a book about the collapse of the English criminal justice system. He was born in Malta in 1951, is a former Trotskyist who, after a spell in the Labour Party, now describes himself as a convinced reactionary. In more than 20 years as a Fleet Street journalist he has been a resident correspondent in both Moscow and Washington and a specialist in education, labour, politics, defence and foreign affairs. He is married with three children.

Tiffany Jenkins is Director of the Arts Programme at the Institute of Ideas. She is the commissioning editor of the society section of the *Debating Matters* series.

Janine Jolly is a health promotion specialist. She has managed young people's health promotion programmes and sexual health promotion programmes. She has also worked for the Sex Education Forum as a Senior Development Officer where she coordinated the Sexual Health in Care Project and the Primary School SRE Project. Janine is co-author of a good practice resource for primary schools.

David J. Landry is Senior Research Associate with The Alan Guttmacher Institute, a non-profit organization specializing in sexual and reproductive health research and public education based in New York and Washington, DC. A demographer and sociologist by training, Landry is co-author of *Sex and America's Teenagers* and has conducted extensive research on sexuality education and sexual behaviour in the United States.

Ellie Lee teaches sociology and social policy at the University of Southampton. Her research interests concern the sociology of social problems and policy developments in the areas of the regulation of reproductive technology and mental health. She is commissioning editor for the law section of the *Debating Matters* series.

Peter Tatchell is a human rights activist, specializing in sexual human rights. For over 30 years, he has championed the cause of queer emancipation with non-violent direct action to challenge homophobia, confronting presidents and archbishops who support discrimination. Articulating a queer agenda that promotes universal sexual freedom, he campaigns for earlier, better quality sex education and for an age of consent of 14 for everyone: gay, straight and bisexual. More of his work can be found at www.petertatchell.net

Stuart Waiton is a community worker, journalist and researcher for the pressure group Generation Youth Issues (www.GenerationYouthIssues.org).

He has spoken at a number of international youth conferences on the importance of an unregulated environment for child and youth development and recently organized a conference in association with Play Scotland on the importance of 'Free Play'. He is researching his doctoral thesis at Glasgow University about the regulation of young people's lives, has written many articles and papers on this subject and is the author of *Scared of the Kids: Curfews, Crime and the Regulation of Young People* (2001).

INTRODUCTION
Ellie Lee and Tiffany Jenkins

The question 'What should schools teach children about sex?' is not a new one. Some sort of sex education has been taught in schools since World War I. Since that time, what knowledge this kind of education aims to impart and to what end, have often been matters of frequently heated debate. This book has been written in recognition, however, that in recent years, sex education has gained a new status and role in education policy compared to the past.

The current legal and policy framework for the provision of sex education, as detailed in the essay in this collection by Simon Blake and Janine Jolly, is complex. As they explain, exactly what schools teach in sex education, and how they teach it, is regulated through a combination of statutory obligations at different stages of the school curriculum, together with policies decided by school governing bodies, in collaboration with parents.

It is clear that the premise behind current policy is that schools should take sex education very seriously indeed. In July 2000 new guidance for schools (entitled *Sex and Relationship Education Guidance*) was issued by the Department for Education and Employment (DfEE). This document was produced in order to address 'uncertainty about what sex and relationship education is and how it should be taught.' It outlines 'good practice' guidelines for head teachers, teachers and school governors and, in doing so, sets out an agenda for the provision of sex education that, according to the Government, is the ideal. The document goes into some detail about both issues of content and teaching practices for sex education. Its overall message, however, is that 'effective sex and relationships education is essential if young people are to make responsible and well-informed decisions about their lives.'

What are the arguments for attaching this degree of importance to sex education? One rationale put forward by the Government is rates of teenage pregnancy in Britain. There is no doubt that New Labour considers teenage pregnancy to be a major social ill. As Tony Blair has argued: 'Britain has the worst record on teenage pregnancies in Europe... As a country we can't afford to ignore this shameful record' (Social Exclusion Unit, *Teenage Pregnancy*, 1999).

While the argument that something must be done about teenage pregnancy in Britain did not emerge first under New Labour (the Conservative Government, in fact, first implemented explicit policy on the issue, through a 1992 White Paper, *The Health of the Nation*), since the late 1990s, policy initiatives on teenage pregnancy have expanded significantly, outstretching anything previously implemented.

In 1999 Tony Blair asked the Social Exclusion Unit, a new team in the Cabinet Office devoted to social problems, to develop an integrated strategy to cut rates of teenage pregnancy and particularly underage parenthood towards the European average. Its report, *Teenage Pregnancy*, was presented to Parliament in June 1999 and it was followed by the establishment of a special government unit, the Teenage Pregnancy Unit, dedicated to this one issue, supported by the Department of Health, of Education and Employment and the Home Office.

It is this report, in part, which laid the way for the new guidance on sex education, published in 2000. In *Teenage Pregnancy*, the role of sex education in schools is ascribed a central, and specific, role. According to the report: 'Research shows that ignorance about sex is a risk factor for teenage pregnancy and that good sex education helps to delay rather than accelerate when young people start sex.' This objective, of delaying the age at which young people start having sex, can be achieved through sex education, since: 'Those who learn about sex mainly from school are less likely to become sexually active under age than those whose family and friends were their main source of support.' The efficacy of school sex education is greater than that achieved through informal contact with friends and family, *Teenage Pregnancy* suggests, since it can help young people deal with 'peer pressure'. 'Young people have to be prepared far more effectively for sex and relationships, ensuring they have the means to deal with the pressure to have sex too soon,' argues the report. The key argument made, in the report's discussion of teenagers' experience of sex, is that teenagers 'are pressured to have sex by their peers, and by a belief that it is expected of them.'

Teenage Pregnancy motivated the need for the new guidance on sex education in schools on this basis; this guidance, to replace that issued for schools in 1994, was necessary to deal with the 'weaknesses in the way schools and families educate young people about sex and relationships. Young people must be better prepared so that they can resist the pressures to have sex too young, deal with emotions and relationships, and use contraception if they do have sex.'

If one key argument for sex education in schools is rates of teenage pregnancy, it is also the case that this kind of education is considered to have a much broader role to play. The objective of the new policy on sex education is not simply to help young people avoid having sex 'too early' and educate them about the importance of using contraception. Its aim is a wider one, of shaping how young people relate to others around them – the use of the term 'sex and relationships education' is in this regard deliberate. As the guidance document puts it: 'Sex and relationships education should contribute to promoting the spiritual, moral, cultural, mental and physical development of pupils at school and of society and preparing pupils for the opportunities, responsibilities and experiences of adult life.'

This broadness of objective is also made clear in the placing of sex and relationships education in the framework of education about 'personal, social and health education' (PSHE) and 'citizenship'. The educational strands that PSHE and citizenship are organized around are: developing confidence and responsibility and making the most of abilities; preparation for playing an active role as a citizen; developing a healthier lifestyle; and developing good relationships and respecting the differences between people. Education to achieve these aims runs from primary school onwards. The delivery of sex and relationships education, states the DfEE guidance, should run in tandem with PSHE through which 'young people learn to respect themselves and others and move with confidence from childhood through adolescence into adulthood.' Sex and relationships education is, therefore, considered to be part of a package of initiatives delivered through schools, through which young people can learn to deal with what might by some be considered 'problems of living'. The framework as a whole intends to 'help pupils develop the skills and understanding they need to live confident, healthy and independent lives.' In this approach, this kind of education is considered as vital a function for schools as teaching conventional subjects, such as maths and English.

Sex and relationships education, then, in the terms of current government policy, is considered to have a key role to play in shaping the behaviour and attitudes of young people, broadly conceived, and those of future generations. There are three key elements to this educational goal, which are summarized in the guidance document as follows:

1 *Attitudes and values*
   - Learning the importance of values and individual conscience and moral considerations.
   - Learning the value of family life, marriage and stable and loving relationships for the nurture of children.
   - Learning the value of respect, love and care.
   - Exploring, considering and understanding moral dilemmas.
   - Developing critical thinking as part of decision making.

2 *Personal and social skills*
   - Learning to manage emotions based on an understanding of difference and with an absence of prejudice.
   - Developing an appreciation of the consequences of choices made.
   - Managing conflict.
   - Learning how to recognize and avoid exploitation and abuse.

3 *Knowledge and understanding*
   - Learning and understanding physical development at appropriate stages.
   - Understanding human sexuality, reproduction, sexual health, emotions and relationships.
   - Learning about contraception and the range of local and national sexual health advice, contraception and support services.

- Learning the reasons for delaying sexual activity and the benefits to be gained from such delay.
- The avoidance of unplanned pregnancy.

This approach to sex education in schools raises a number of questions that this book seeks to address. Can sex and relationships education lead to a reduction in rates of teenage pregnancy and STIs (sexually transmitted infections)? Is the relationship between knowledge taught in schools about sex and relationships and the age at which young people have sex as policy makers envisage it to be? Can schools significantly improve the ability of young people to develop positive relationships with others? If the aim of sex and relationships education is to equip young people for adult life, is the balance currently envisaged between schools and other social institutions, such as the family, the right one? In sum, is the current direction of sex education policy addressing the right problems and offering the right solutions? The aim of this volume is to offer readers the opportunity to consider competing responses to these questions.

The first essay offers a perspective from the United States, as a point of comparison to the debate and policy developments in Britain. Authored by David J. Landry of the USA-based research organization, The Alan Guttmacher Institute, this essay focuses on the problems that may be posed by approaches to sex education that encourage young people to just 'say no' to sex. In the USA, reports Landry, abstinence-only programmes have gained ground in some states in North America since 1996. Such programmes advocate that since 'true love waits', sex should take place only within marriage and only by abstaining until this point, can young people truly avoid the health risks associated with sexual activity. Landry makes a strong case against such programmes, on the grounds that they are unrealistic in a society where the age of marriage is steadily rising and where it is simply not the case that people remain monogamous through married life. This essay points to the practical pitfalls associated with policies that presuppose it is possible to discourage young people from having sex at all in their teenage years.

Landry makes the point that school-based sex education in the USA is primarily justified on public health grounds, those of teenage pregnancy prevention and reducing rates of infection from sexually transmitted infection. The essay that follows, by Simon Blake and Janine Jolly of the Sex Education Forum, indicates that in Britain an additional justification has emerged – that of assisting young people in developing (personal and social skills). They argue for sex *and* relationships education, defined as 'lifelong learning about sex, sexuality, emotions, relationships and sexual health.' Sex and relationships education, for Blake and Jolly, aims not only to reduce rates of pregnancy and STIs in young people, but also to help them acquire a range of skills that can equip them for developing relationships with others. These contributors argue that a crucial rationale for this approach is that this is the kind of sex education young people, not just policy makers, say they want.

While Blake and Jolly's essay suggests that current government policy is moving in broadly the right direction, the next three essays raise criticisms of contrasting kinds of sex education in Britain today. Community worker and researcher Stuart Waiton is particularly critical of the idea, central to current government thinking, that the problem for young people is of pressure to have sex 'too early'. He takes issue first with so-called 'evidence-based' grounds for the problematization of teenage sex, those of rates of teenage pregnancy and of STIs. In contrast to the current orthodoxy, Waiton contends that neither is a major social problem. Panic about rates of HIV infection and of chlamydia is unwarranted, rates of pregnancy in under-16s are not increasing and a figure of only 3,700 births per year in this age group does not justify the high profile of the teenage pregnancy 'problem', he argues. Waiton's case is not only that sex and relationships education is unjustified on health grounds, but that it may be damaging for young people. The vogue for presenting peer group relationships as a problem, that necessitate young people being guided by sex educators about how to relate to their friends is, for Waiton, the real cause for concern. This approach, he argues, is depriving young people of the chance to experiment and learn for themselves how to relate to others – a process that it is vital for them to engage in, free from adult interference.

The final two essays, by journalist Peter Hitchens and human rights activist Peter Tatchell, both criticize sex education as currently practised, but from polar points of view. For Hitchens, sex education has been a manifest failure. It has contributed to, not alleviated, all the problems it purports to solve – for example, rates of STIs and teenage pregnancy. It has done so because it has amplified, not diminished, the sexualization of culture and society, through which innocence has been made impossible and degrading images of sex and promiscuous behaviour prevail. In this context, moral sense – the ability to distinguish between right and wrong in sexual behaviour and personal life – has been almost destroyed. At the centre of this demoralization of society, argues Hitchens, lies an attack on marriage and the family. 'Progressive' campaigners have, over the past century, waged a concerted war against the family and in favour of the state. The argument for sex education in schools has been a central aspect of this campaign and, to the detriment of children and society as a whole, it has succeeded. Sex education is the culprit of the piece for Hitchens and only a determined effort to make a wholly unapologetic case for the moral importance of marriage and family life can save the day.

An entirely different sense of the problem of sex education today is communicated through Peter Tatchell's contribution. The problem, argues Tatchell, is not that sex is discussed too overtly with young people, but that it is not discussed overtly enough. 'Sex lessons,' argues Tatchell 'should tell the truth: sex is good for us. It is natural, wholesome, fun and healthy.' Nothing should be off bounds for discussion – all sexual practices should be discussed with young people in schools if they are curious about them – including anal and oral sex. Sex education should move away from its current presentation of sex as dangerous and harmful and, instead, tackle the risk of STIs and pregnancy and promote safer sex as a glamorous and enjoyable activity. Such 'sexing up' of sex education does not, however, for this author imply a loss of moral sense. Rather, he contends, such sex education can promote a highly moral attitude towards relationships, based not on outmoded concepts of the superiority of marriage and conventional family, but on those of mutual respect, concern and fulfilment.

So what should we teach children about sex? While this book does not present straightforward answers to this question, we hope the essays that follow debate this contentious issue in a thought-provoking and intelligent way.

Essay One

SEX EDUCATION: A VIEW FROM THE UNITED STATES
David J. Landry

A number of important studies and controversies related to school-based sex education have emerged in the United States over the past several years. Lessons from the USA could inform the debate in the UK over school-based sex education, both in terms of approaches to follow, as well as ones to avoid. Similarly, if the USA could adapt some of the examples of sexuality education and services developed in Western Europe, teenage pregnancy in America would likely be at a much lower rate.

In the United States the most contentious debate over sexuality education is between comprehensive approaches and abstinence-only-until-marriage strategies. Comprehensive programmes usually cover how young people can develop skills to delay the onset of sexual intercourse, but they also provide information on how persons can reduce the risk of STIs (sexually transmitted infections) and pregnancy when they do become sexually active. In contrast, abstinence-until-marriage programmes emphasize that all sexual activity outside of the context of marriage is unhealthy and unacceptable, generally information on contraception is either not discussed at all or failure rates are emphasized. There is an array of less extreme abstinence programmes that do not necessarily require that young people abstain until marriage. Some abstinence programmes even cover contraception in a more balanced way. But the most aggressive and visible promoters of abstinence, only countenance abstinence-only-until-marriage.

In this essay I briefly review the latest statistics on teenage pregnancy in the United States; highlight views of the general public, parents, sex education teachers and students on their beliefs about sex education; discuss some approaches to school-based sex education that have been demonstrated to be successful; review findings on the actual content of sex education in the United States; discuss the rise of the abstinence-only-until-marriage movement; and finally discuss the future of sexuality education in the United States.

TEENAGE PREGNANCY AND STIs IN THE UNITED STATES

In the United States support for school-based sexuality education is usually promoted principally on public health grounds related to preventing high rates of teenage pregnancy and STIs. Indeed, a review of recent trends in the United States demonstrates the gravity of the situation. For instance, while many have celebrated that the teenage pregnancy rate has been declining since 1992, the USA still has one of the highest rates in the industrialized world. In 1996, the latest year comparable figures are available internationally, the USA had a teenage pregnancy rate of 97 per 1,000. This rate is twice as high as England and Wales or Canada and nine times higher than Japan or the Netherlands. As a consequence, each year, almost one million teenage women – or about ten per cent of all women aged 15–19 in the United States – become pregnant. More than four in ten women still get pregnant before the age of 20. A full 78 per cent of these pregnancies are unintended and 56 per cent of them end in birth, 30 per cent in abortion and 14 per cent in miscarriage.

Sexually transmitted diseases also are highly prevalent among US youth. Every year three million teens – about one in four – become infected with an STI. The emergence of HIV/AIDS mobilized many in the USA to educate youth about HIV/AIDS. Many states even passed laws mandating HIV/AIDS education in public schools. The Center for Disease Control and Prevention (CDC) estimates that at least half of all HIV infections in the USA occur among people under the age of 25. While HIV/AIDS was once predominant among men who have sex with men, the epidemic has spread more widely. The CDC estimates that among infected adolescents, the proportion that are female is growing dramatically, perhaps exceeding 50 per cent.

Despite the fact that the USA has high pregnancy and STI rates, sexual activity rates are not particularly higher than in Western European countries. By the age of 17, 52 per cent of females and 59 per cent of males in the USA have had sexual intercourse. By the time these teens are 19 years old, 81 per cent have had sex.

Despite the fact that teenage pregnancy and STIs are at high levels across the United States, the federal government and state-level governments have had relatively little influence over the content of local school-based sex education programmes. An Alan Guttmacher Institute survey of school superintendents found that local sexuality education policies are most influenced by local level actors such as the local school board, the school district superintendent, school principals, curriculum directors, the teachers themselves as well as parents and community members. Traditionally, the federal government has most often been involved in funding model programmes and in providing financial support to a limited number of state and local communities to implement model programmes, demonstration projects and the like. At the state level, states often provide technical guidance and general standards and some provide limited funding to local school districts to implement programmes. As a consequence of localities having considerable control over their sexuality education curriculum the content of sexuality education is often quite varied and uneven across the USA.

THE RISE OF ABSTINENCE-ONLY UNTIL MARRIAGE

The prominence of the federal government's influence on sexuality education policy began to change dramatically with the 1996 welfare reform legislation passed by Congress that guarantees 50 million federal dollars per year until 2002 for abstinence education programmes. In addition, states are required to match every four dollars of these federal funds with three dollars in state or local funds, bringing the expected annual expenditure to $87.5 million. The federal government allocates these funds to states and states then either directly administer the funds or provide grants to other public agencies or to private non-profit agencies. A significant proportion of these funds are used for school-based abstinence-only until-marriage education. To qualify for federal funding education programmes must adhere to an eight-point definition of abstinence. Taken as a whole, the definition is so extreme that it bears quoting in its entirety. Recipients of the funding must ensure their programme:

1 has as its exclusive purpose, teaching the social, psychological and health gains to be realized by abstaining from sexual activity
2 teaches abstinence from sexual activity outside marriage as the expected standard for all school-age children
3 teaches that abstinence from sexual activity is the only certain way to avoid out of wedlock pregnancy, sexually transmitted diseases and other associated health problems
4 teaches that a mutually faithful monogamous relationship in context of marriage is the expected standard of human sexual activity

5 teaches that sexual activity outside the context of marriage is likely to have harmful psychological and physical effects

6 teaches that bearing children out of wedlock is likely to have harmful consequences for the child, the child's parents and society

7 teaches young people how to reject sexual advances and how alcohol and drug use increases vulnerability to sexual advances

8 teaches the importance of attaining self-sufficiency before engaging in sexual activity.

(Source: P. L. 104–193, section 401a)

By their success in codifying these beliefs (some with no scientific basis) into law, the religious right gave their abstinence-only-until-marriage movement greater visibility and a broader stamp of legitimacy. The main reason the religious right vigorously opposes comprehensive sexuality education is that it teaches young persons that they should use contraception if they are sexually active. The religious right in America is on a crusade to uphold their version of 'traditional family values'. They believe sexual activity outside the context of marriage is a great threat to the traditional family. They also vigorously oppose other movements, trends and services that they view as threats to 'traditional family values' such as the women's movement, gay liberation, multiculturalism, cohabitation, confidential health services for minors and abortion. Institutional support for alternative family and household forms, such as single parent families, gay families and cohabiting couples are strongly opposed by the religious right.

The religious right approaches the abstinence message with a missionary zeal. They want to impose their moral code, or their version of 'traditional family values', on all Americans. To restore the family, unwed teens and young adults, gays and lesbians and even widowed and divorced persons must abstain from all sexual activity. Their goal is to create a culture where sex is permissible only within the context of a legal marriage between a man and a woman.

The abstinence-only-until-marriage movement is becoming more sophisticated over time. In the past, some abstinence advocates aggressively promoted the idea that HIV could permeate latex condoms. When this claim was discredited, to better confront public health oriented advocates, abstinence-until-marriage advocates began to make more scientific and factually based arguments. Relatively new organizations such as the Physicians Consortium and the Medical Institute for Sexual Health have adopted public health style scientific analyses by medical professionals from an abstinence perspective. To discourage sex outside marriage, they now emphasize user failure rates of contraception and STI incidence statistics. They generally do not discuss how user failure rates can be reduced by better and more consistent use.

◆ ● ●
● ● **SUPPORT FOR SCHOOL-BASED SEXUALITY**
● ● ◆ **EDUCATION IN THE UNITED STATES**

Representative surveys of adults in the USA reflect that the public favours a gradual, age-appropriate, comprehensive and factual approach to sexuality education. The vast majority of parents want abstinence from sex emphasized, but they also want their children to have information on how to prevent STIs and pregnancy for when they are sexually active. For instance, a series of Kaiser Family Foundation surveys, released in a report titled *Sex Education in America,* demonstrated that there is widespread support for comprehensive sexuality education. Almost all parents, 94 per cent, wanted schools to address such issues as pressure to have sex and the emotional consequences of becoming sexually active. Over 80 per cent of parents say how to use condoms and other forms of birth control, as well as how to talk about them with partners, should be taught in the schools. Over three-quarters thought controversial topics such as abortion, and sexual orientation should be discussed. A 1999 public opinion poll of over 1,000 adults across the United States, sponsored by Advocates for Youth and the Sexuality Information and Education and Council of the United States (SIECUS), showed more than 80 per cent of Americans believe young people should be given information on how to protect themselves from unplanned pregnancy and STIs, as well as about abstinence.

THE CONTENT OF SEX EDUCATION

ABSTINENCE

In part, to ascertain the inroads of the abstinence-only movement on school-based sexuality education, The Alan Guttmacher Institute conducted a survey of US public sexuality education teachers in 1999 that was similar to one they conducted 11 years earlier. In 1988 only two per cent of teachers stated that they presented abstinence as the only way to prevent STIs and pregnancy. By 1999 that proportion had grown to 23 per cent. While a full 60 per cent of sexuality education teachers emphasized the effectiveness of contraceptive methods, 28 per cent emphasized the ineffectiveness of condoms in preventing STIs and/or the ineffectiveness of birth control in preventing pregnancy. An additional 12 per cent did not cover birth control or condom use at all.

OTHER TOPICS

As with parents and the general public, over 80 per cent of sexuality education teachers support teaching about birth control, abortion and sexual orientation, but the percentage actually teaching these topics steeply declined between 1988 and 1999. Fewer students are receiving information on key sexuality education topics today compared to a decade ago. For instance, while in 1988, a full 92 per cent of sexuality education teachers covered birth control methods by the twelfth grade (students aged 17 to 18), in 1999 only 77 per cent did. Sexual orientation was covered by 69 per cent of teachers in 1988, but only by 51 per cent in 1999.

There are large gaps between the high percentage of teachers recommending that topics should be taught and the lower percentage of teachers that actually cover those topics. For instance, 89 per cent of teachers felt information on where to go for birth control should be covered by the twelfth grade but only 65 per cent actually covered it in any grade. The gap on other topics such as ethical and factual information about abortion, the correct way to use a condom and sexual orientation is large – between 24 and 30 percentage points.

Other studies confirm that school-based sexuality education occurs too late in the United States. According to an Urban Institute study, while some sort of sexuality education was received by virtually all students by the time they completed high school, a full 30 per cent of males (and 46 per cent of black males) aged 15-19 did not receive any formal sex education before they first had sex.

While virtually all students are learning skills in how to abstain from sexual intercourse, many students, particularly those in abstinence-only programmes, are only learning skills related to resisting sex. They are much less likely to learn about how to reduce their risk if they are sexually active by covering such topics as partner communication, how to access sexual and reproductive health services and the importance of using contraception correctly and consistently.

◈ ● ● MYTHS OF SEXUALITY EDUCATION DISPELLED

THE MYTH THAT PROGRAMMES ARE NOT EFFECTIVE

In May 2000 the National Campaign to Prevent Teenage Pregnancy (hereafter the Campaign), a non-profit organization that includes both conservative and liberal advocates of sexuality education, released the report *Emerging Answers: Research Findings on Programs to Reduce Teen Pregnancy*. The report analysed the findings from rigorously evaluated teenage pregnancy prevention programmes in the United States.

The report documented the characteristics of programmes that were proven to successfully delay the onset of sex, reduce the frequency of sex, reduce the numbers of partners among teens, increase the use of condoms and other forms of contraception and reduce teen pregnancy. Some encouraging results included that the strength of the evidence for the effectiveness of sex and HIV education programmes have increased significantly during recent years. Moreover, the effects of programmes have been found to be more lasting than prior evaluations of older programmes. The report also found, however, that there is no conclusive evidence that abstinence-only programmes are effective. The report noted that many abstinence-only programmes have not been subjected to scientifically rigorous evaluations. Despite the large federal and state investment in abstinence-only programmes, results from a federally funded effort to evaluate several abstinence-only programmes are not expected for over a year.

A CDC-sponsored review of several evaluated sexuality education programmes also found positive impacts among school-based programmes in reducing the rate of initiation to sexual intercourse, increasing communication with parents about abstinence and contraception, increasing acceptance of condoms among participants, reducing the number of partners students had sex with and increasing contraceptive use among those that did have intercourse. The Campaign review of programmes that work and do not work found that, among other factors, to be successful programmes must: be of significant duration to be effective; deliver and consistently reinforce a clear accurate message about ways to avoid intercourse and use methods of protection against pregnancy and STIs when sexually active; incorporate behavioural goals; and use teaching methods and materials that are appropriate to the age, sexual experience and culture of the students.

THE MYTH THAT SEX EDUCATION PROMOTES SEXUAL ACTIVITY

Many conservatives have attacked comprehensive sexuality education programmes by claiming that teaching about contraception will promote sexual activity among youth who otherwise would abstain. A similar argument states that a dual message, that it is best to abstain, but if you are sexually active use contraception, is confusing to teenagers. Yet the Campaign report noted: 'The overwhelming weight of evidence shows that sex education that discusses contraception does not hasten the onset of sex, increase the frequency of sex, nor increase the number of sexual partners.' In fact, several of the studies cited in the report do the opposite: they delay sex and increase contraceptive use. The report went on to conclude that 'making condoms or other contraceptives available in schools does not hasten or increase sexual activity.' Even the general public disagrees with this myth that sexuality education promotes sex. The Advocates for Youth/SIECUS poll showed a full 78 per cent of the population rejects the idea that providing sexuality education encourages sexual activity.

THE MYTH THAT ABSTINENCE IS THE ONLY 100 PER CENT SAFE METHOD

When abstinence fails the consequences can be severe. In the United States the Southern Baptist Church has organized over two-and-a-half million adolescents to take a public virginity pledge where they promised to abstain from sex until marriage. A thorough analysis of the impact of the virginity pledge by the sociologists Bearman and Brückner showed that adolescents who took the pledge were much less likely to have intercourse. But they confirmed a fear that many people have of abstinence-only programmes. When the pledgers did have sex they were less likely to use contraception at first intercourse. The authors conclude 'that pledgers, like other adolescents, would benefit from knowledge about contraception and pregnancy risk, even if they think at the time they do not need such knowledge.' The research also showed virginity pledges work only in specific contexts, in particular, they can be effective among younger adolescents who represent a moral community that is less than 40 per cent of their school population. When pledgers constitute a larger proportion of the student body the effect becomes negative.

WHY ABSTINENCE UNTIL MARRIAGE IS AN UNREALISTIC NATIONAL POLICY

The abstinence-until-marriage movement's expected standard of behaviour is simple: Abstain from all sexual activity until marriage, then marry someone who has also abstained from sex and have a monogamous marriage. Abstinence-only until marriage advocates state this is the one true safe sex strategy to avoid STIs and unintended pregnancy. While most Americans see nothing wrong with people who aspire to this type of behaviour, most believe that to make this a social policy for every American to follow is simply unrealistic. Indeed, it would take nothing less than divine intervention to reverse the social trends that prevent all Americans from following this standard of conduct.

Most in the abstinence-until-marriage movement vaguely portray the period of abstinence as ending sometime shortly after the teen years. But in the United States the age at first marriage has been steadily rising since the 1970s. In 2000, the age at which half of men and women first married (or the median age at marriage) was 25.1 and 26.8 respectively. Moreover, a significant a proportion of men and women remain unmarried into their thirties. For instance, by age 30.9, 25 per cent of women in the United States have still not married.

While it may be safer to marry a partner who has never had sex, the effort to find one may further delay age at marriage. The abstinence-until-marriage movement simply fails to take into account the scope of sexual activity in our society. Currently the median age of first intercourse in the United States is 16.9 for men and 17.4 for women. By 21 years of age, 90 per cent of men and women have had intercourse. In fact only 22 per cent of women aged 18–59 and 10 per cent of men waited until they were married to first have intercourse.

If a young person succeeds in remaining abstinent until marriage and finding a partner who has done so, a remaining challenge is for the couple to remain mutually monogamous throughout life. The first uncomfortable fact is that about 50 per cent of American marriages end in divorce. But even if a couple remains married there are risks. Over 30 per cent of pregnancies among married adults in the United States are unintended (this is one reason why contraceptive sterilization is the leading method of birth control in the USA). About 25 per cent of men and 15 per cent of women have reported that they have had an extramarital affair. Moreover it is estimated at any one time a full 10 per cent of married women in the United States are at risk of STIs because either they have multiple partners or their husband has another partner.

Those who can fulfill the abstinence until marriage social contract have earned my respect, but it is hardly a national model for all Americans. Dan Savage, a widely syndicated advice columnist, took safer sex practices to their logical extreme in responding to a reader who stated that his life example of abstinence-until-marriage was the only true method of safe sex. Savage replied: 'The only way to truly avoid STIs and unplanned pregnancies and heartaches and breakups and divorce is to never have sex at all – casual or marital. If eliminating any risk of contracting STDs is your objective, I'd advise you to divorce the wife and have yourself castrated.'

THE FUTURE OF SEXUALITY EDUCATION IN THE UNITED STATES

The political tactics of the religious right regarding sexuality education keep becoming more extreme. After a change in the presidential administration, and several months of delays, in summer 2001 the Surgeon General of the United States released the report *The Surgeon General's Call to Action to Promote Sexual Health and Responsible Sexual Behavior*. While the report is groundbreaking in several respects, the Surgeon General had to go to great lengths to defend school-based sex education. For instance, the report noted that: 'Parents are the primary educators and should guide a child's sexuality in a way consistent with their values and beliefs. They also recognize that families differ in their level of knowledge and comfort in discussing such issues, making school education a vital component in providing equity of access to information.' Despite the relatively cautious language and an abstinence promotion message the report attracted severe criticism among many of those opposed to comprehensive sex education. One conservative news release read: 'A coalition of pro-family organizations expressed outrage over the Surgeon General's report... that promotes sexual diseases and irresponsible behavior.' Many observers thought that the report would never be released after the Bush administration took over the White House. While President Bush has allowed the report to be issued, he has not endorsed it. In fact, after the report was released President Bush's administration reaffirmed his support of abstinence-only-until marriage education. Given that the President is unlikely to give the report much support, future federal action based on the reports findings are uncertain at best.

Conservatives continue to keep government representatives off balance and in a retreat from positions that might support comprehensive sexuality education. In an effort to persuade young people that they should stop having sex until they are in a married, a coalition of conservatives are attempting to discredit safer sex practices by questioning the effectiveness of condoms against many STIs. When the CDC released a report in July 2000 on the efficacy of condoms in STI prevention, the religious right responded by organizing a very public effort to force the resignation of the director of the CDC (the effort has so far failed).

We have proven strategies to teach students how to abstain from sex and reduce the risk of pregnancy and STIs when they do become sexually active. The challenge is to continue to implement and replicate the success of these programmes. Another challenge is to continue to refine these approaches as well as to explore other promising approaches. Clearly school-based sexuality education programmes alone are not sufficient. If parent-child communication, community programmes, media messages and the healthcare system are able to deliver a more consistent message about abstinence pregnancy and STI prevention then we will be more likely to see positive outcomes. A country on one end of the spectrum, the Netherlands, comes the closest to achieving this ideal and as a result they have among the lowest rates of teenage pregnancy and STIs in the industrialized world. By way of contrast, the United States is divided on what its message to youth should be.

Those promoting abstinence-only-until-marriage are not satisfied that their own children receive such education. They want to impose their standard of behaviour on Americans who support more comprehensive approaches. The divide may never be closed. While respecting those who want their children to have an abstinence-until-marriage education, as adults we have a responsibility to provide students with the environment where they can learn vital information. Parents and educators need our support in helping their children and students become healthy adults. Young people need information that is accurate and balanced, so that they can make informed choices and protect themselves.

Suggested websites for further information about sexuality education in the United States

The Alan Guttmacher Institute: www.agi-usa.org

The National Abstinence Clearinghouse: www.abstinence.net

The National Campaign to Prevent Teenage Pregnancy: www.teenpregnancy.org

The Kaiser Family Foundation: www.kff.org

The Sexuality Information and Education Council of the United States: www.siecus.org

---

Essay Two

EVIDENCE AND ENTITLEMENT: TEACHING ABOUT SEX AND RELATIONSHIPS IN SCHOOLS

Simon Blake and Janine Jolly

Sex and relationships education remains one of the most politicized areas of the school curriculum. Moral and political rhetoric about what we should teach children at what age, how they should be taught and where they should be taught continues to permeate political, media and public debate. In the UK, as in the United States, there is a small but effective lobby that vociferously opposes sex and relationships education in schools. Their argument is based on a number of beliefs. These include that by teaching children and young people about sex and relationships we encourage them to have sex earlier; that sex and relationships education is taught without a values framework, and that sex and relationships education should be the role of parents not schools. It is also based on the belief that young people are not good decision makers and therefore we need to make decisions for them. This prevents children and young people from receiving their entitlement to good-quality sex and relationships education. It undermines teacher confidence to deliver sex and relationships education and it disregards the considerable evidence base from both here and abroad that timely, well-thought through sex and relationships education, delivered by trained and confident educators, can delay the onset of sexual activity, as well as ensure that young people are more likely to behave responsibly when they do become sexually active.

Young people themselves continually report that the sex and relationships education they receive is too late, too narrow and too biological in focus; in short, it fails to address their needs and concerns. Therefore the question is not: Should we or shouldn't we talk about sex and relationships with children and young people? Neither is it: What should we teach them? But instead we should ask: When are we going to genuinely to listen to young people and ensure that we offer them what they need? And how are we going to ensure that children and young people get the sex and relationships education they need and deserve?

WHAT IS SEX AND RELATIONSHIP EDUCATION?

An important step forward for sex education was the establishment of the Sex Education Forum, based at the National Children's Bureau. The Forum is a unique collaboration of 50 organizations including religious, health, education, children's, parenting and specialist organizations. Established in 1987, following new legislation affecting sex and relationships education, the Forum aims to promote sex and relationships education for all children and young people at home; in school and educational settings; and in health, youth, community and public care settings. The objectives of the Forum are to stimulate informed public debate in sex and relationships education; support parents, teachers, school governors, youth workers, social workers, health professionals, head teachers, senior managers and others by gathering and disseminating information about new initiatives, research, methodology, resources and support services; and encourage appropriate initial and in-service training of all those involved. Since 1999, the Forum has defined sex and relationships education as lifelong learning about sex, sexuality, emotions, relationships and sexual health. It involves acquiring skills and forming positive beliefs, values and attitudes.

TOWARDS GOOD PRACTICE

The Sex Education Forum members have worked over the past 15 years to define, recognize and support the development of good practice in sex and relationships education. In summary the following key issues emerge. Messages and learning in sex and relationships education need to be supported by a *whole school ethos*. This is essential for effective teaching and learning across the curriculum. An ethos and context that models and experiences positive relationships among teachers, pupils, support staff and the wider community is an essential prerequisite for sex and relationships education. *Training and support* is necessary for high-quality sex and relationships education. Teachers need to feel confident in both the content and methodology for sex and relationships education. They need to feel supported by an effective *sex and relationships policy* that outlines the content, approach and boundaries. The policy should be developed in consultation with *teachers*, *health professionals*, *pupils*, *parents and the wider community* and include a clear and explicit *values framework* that all teachers will work within. Sex and relationships education should form part of an *overall personal, social and health education and citizenship programme* that is underpinned by the promotion of *emotional resourcefulness and self-esteem.* Sex and relationships education needs to consist of three clear elements, *knowledge, skills and attitudes and values* and use *active learning methods* that engage children and young people in the learning process. School-based sex and relationships should be well connected to *sexual health* and *advice services.* The programme should meet the needs of all pupils, *boys as well as girls*, those who are *lesbian and gay*, those with *special needs* and *people from different ethnicities and faiths*. All sex and relationships education should be *monitored and assessed* to ensure learning. It needs to be *developmental and progressive*, building on what they have learnt before and be mindful of the diversity of experience within the classroom.

◆ ● ●
● ●
● ● ◆ **THE CURRENT PICTURE**

England currently has the highest rate of teenage pregnancy in Western Europe (Social Exclusion Unit, *Teenage Pregnancy*, 1999) and, according to a Public Health Laboratory Report published in 2000, rising rates of sexually transmitted infections (STIs).

THE LEGAL AND POLICY FRAMEWORK

School sex and relationships education forms part of the National Curriculum in Science in both primary and secondary school. This focuses on the reproductive aspects of sex. In secondary schools there is also a legal requirement to provide, as a minimum, information about sexually transmitted infections (STIs) including HIV. All other aspects of sex and relationships education, including the broader aspects about relationships and values, are left to the discretion of the governing body of the school. The *Sex and Relationships Education Guidance* from the Department for Education and Employment (DfEE) (2000) does, however, emphasize the importance of addressing skills development and values exploration. Schools need to feel better supported in meeting the needs of children and young people so that they can confidently address the broader aspects of sex and relationships education including communication skills, negotiation skills, assertiveness and positive self-esteem. Recent developments within education have gone some way to enable this process although, as they are not statutory, arguably they have not gone far enough.

The *National Curriculum Handbooks for Primary and Secondary Schools* (QCA/DfEE, 1999) highlight the role of schools in ensuring that pupils are able to develop their knowledge and understanding of their own and different beliefs within an equal opportunities framework. It also highlights the role of schools in promoting pupils' self-esteem and emotional well being and helping them to form and maintain satisfying relationships. Sex and relationships education as part of a broad-based personal, social and health education (PSHE) programme is central to achieving this.

There are aspects of sex and relationships education in the National Curriculum Science Order that children and young people must receive. In addition, governors are responsible for developing a policy that describes what is offered outside the science curriculum. Primary schools can decide not to provide anything outside science but must have a policy statement that states whether and what they provide. However, the *Sex and Relationship Education Guidance* recommends: 'that all primary schools should have a sex and relationships education programme tailored to the age and the physical and emotional maturity of the children.' Secondary schools are required to provide a sex and relationships programme that includes, as a minimum, information about sexually transmitted infections including HIV/AIDS.

The *National Curriculum for Schools* (QCA/DfEE, 2000) now includes a non-statutory framework for PSHE and citizenship at primary school. At secondary level PSHE remains non-statutory and citizenship will be statutory from September 2002 (*National Curriculum Handbook for Secondary Schools*, QCA/DfEE, 1999). These frameworks provide a planning tool for schools to deliver PSHE and citizenship across all key stages for children and young people aged five to 16. There are four strands: developing confidence and responsibility and making the most of their abilities; preparing to play an active role as citizens; developing a healthy safer lifestyle; and developing good relationships and respecting the differences between people.

This overall framework provides a planning tool for schools to think about what they should be delivering in sex and relationships education as part of a broad based PSHE and citizenship programme. To support the PSHE and citizenship framework, there is additional guidance through the guidelines from the DfEE in *Sex and Relationship Education Guidance*. This is supported in legislation by the Learning and Skills Act (2000). This Act requires that young people learn about the nature of marriage and its importance for family life and the bringing up of children and are protected from teaching and materials which are inappropriate, having regard to the age and religious and cultural background of the pupils concerned.

ADDRESSING DIVERSITY – SPECIFIC ISSUES IN THE DFEE SEX AND RELATIONSHIP EDUCATION GUIDANCE

Sex and relationships education has a role in challenging prejudice and homophobia and supporting the acceptance and valuing of diversity. In developing sex and relationships education for children and young people, schools will need to pay careful attention to diversity. As with all other parts of the curriculum, sex and relationships education should support *all* children and young people. Educators need the confidence to incorporate diversity into the whole of the sex and relationships programme, not to see it as an adjunct that can be addressed in one lesson or excluded all together.

The *Sex and Relationship Education Guidance* from the DfEE highlights a number of key issues that need to be considered in the planning and delivery of sex and relationships education. *A focus on the needs of boys as well as girls* is important. The context and expectations of boys and girls is different from how it was two decades ago. Social, cultural and economic changes have meant that gender roles are more fluid and changing. Boys and young men often feel excluded on the basis of its narrow reproductive focus and disengage from sex and relationships education. This narrow reproductive focus is not good enough for girls either. Both girls and boys need opportunities to explore gender roles, expectations, hopes and fears as well as learning about sexuality, relationships and all aspects of sexual health including contraception and safer sex.

An understanding of faith, culture and ethnicity needs to inform sex and relationships education content and delivery. Values and norms in sex and relationships education need to be reflective of the diversity within British culture and children need opportunities to explore and think about different sexual and cultural values. *Children with special needs* may need extra sex and relationships education that is well planned, coordinated and delivered to meet their particular needs. The approach and methodology may need to be different but the principles of openness and entitlement remain the same. Sex and relationships education can play a role in preventing the abuse of these particularly vulnerable children and young people. Children and young people with a *gay or lesbian sexual identity and orientation* need access to education that is relevant to them. Very often sex and relationships education excludes the needs of gay and lesbian young people.

HOW DO CHILDREN LEARN ABOUT SEX?

From a very early age children are learning about sex and receiving messages about sex and relationships. These messages about sex, gender and sexuality begin almost as soon as we are born. We are surrounded by them. Like most other things that humans learn about, information comes from a range of sources. Children gain information in a way that is a little bit like a jigsaw puzzle – they get one piece here and another piece there. Sometimes the pieces fit, sometimes they do not and muddles are compounded if children feel unable to ask questions and clarify what they think they know. Children learn from both formal and informal sources, family and friends; the media; theatre, at school and in the youth club; at the doctors and other health settings. Some of the messages are positive and helpful. Too often they are not. They learn from a very early age about gender and sexuality by the clothes boys and girls are dressed in and the toys they are encouraged to play with. Comics and magazines impart messages about gender roles, sex and sexuality. They learn from both implicit and explicit messages. Children also learn by watching and observing the relationships and the way adults behave with each other. Silence and embarrassment, violence and disrespect, provide equally strong messages as the spoken word.

As children grow up they piece this information together consciously and unconsciously. Depending on the messages and the approach, these pieces can form a rich mosaic or a gloomy picture. In Britain we still have an uncomfortable culture where it is difficult to talk about sex and relationships in a sensible way. Instead we can rely on smut and innuendo to communicate about sex and sexuality. This is not helpful to children and young people. It results in their growing up knowing only myths and misinformation, learnt from the playground or from television. Too many children grow up scared and confused, worried that they are not normal or that there is something wrong with them. Too many children grow up unconfident or unsure, without the understanding and skills they need to form positive relationships and manage their sexual health. This needs to change.

WHAT DO CHILDREN AND YOUNG PEOPLE SAY THEY WANT?

The Sex Education Forum is committed to listening to the views and wants of children and young people. Too often their views are left out in matters concerning them. Time and again they tell us that their sex and relationships education is not good enough. They tell us it focuses on the biological aspects of reproduction, happens too late to be helpful, so they often get sex and relationships education after they have experienced puberty, after they experience sexual attraction and after they have had sexual experiences. This clearly does not help or support them.

At a consultation event with young people, the Forum made a video, *Please Minister, can we have better sex and relationships education*? and a charter that were sent to David Blunkett, then Secretary of State for Education. In these, young people outlined their desire for sex and relationships education that started early, was fun, delivered by well-trained and experienced educators, addressed different sexualities and engaged them in classroom learning activities where they can learn from discussions and problem solving. They particularly emphasized that as well as information they want opportunities to develop personal and social skills within role-play, discussion and other learning activities. They also want to explore what they describe as real life dilemmas, such as when to have sex and how to be yourself in a relationship.

Their charter demonstrates that young people have a whole range of ideas for improving their sex and relationships education and we could do well to listen to them in among the other voices.

our charter
for good sex and
relationships education

⇨ every child has the right to sex education in all areas
(gay, lesbian, straight, bisexual)
⇨ every child has the right to express their opinion
⇨ every child has the right to specific information, advice, counselling and support

to achieve this ...

- We want Society to be more open about sex in general
- Parents should be able to talk to their children without feeling embarrassed
- There should be a special sex education team
- Teachers who feel comfortable to give sex education should be given support, courses and workshops
- Outside visitors should be allowed to come into schools

we would expect to learn about ...

- Real-life dilemmas
- Sexuality and relationship issues:
  - peer pressure
  - problems
  - friendships
  - being gay or lesbian
  - contraception
  - STIs
  - HIV
- Pros and cons about sex
  - when is the right time to have sex?
  - where to go and get advice (eg Brook)
- We would like free booklets to take away

we would like sex education to be fun ...

This would be through:
- role plays and games
- videos
- opportunities to explore dilemmas
- practising communication
- discussions that are open and multi-ethnic
- comments and suggestions box allowing pupils to ask questions who would otherwise feel embarrassed and gives us a chance to say what we want to know
- using mechanical baby dolls

we would like outside visitors to come and talk to us ...

- teenage mothers
- a lesbian or gay man
- people with different life experiences to express
- people from clinics

SEX
EDUCATION
FORUM

This Charter was written by young people attending a
National Children's Bureau Talkshop event on 26 February 2000.

◆ ● ●
● ● **A FRAMEWORK FOR SEX AND**
● ● ◆ **RELATIONSHIPS EDUCATION**

The Sex Education Forum believes that sex and relationships education should be an integral part of the lifelong learning process, beginning in early childhood and continuing into adult life. It should be an entitlement for all children, young people and adults and should meet the needs of boys as well as girls; those who are heterosexual, lesbian, gay or bisexual; those with physical, learning or emotional difficulties; and those with a religious or faith tradition. It needs to encourage personal and social development fostering self-esteem, self-awareness, a sense of moral responsibility and the confidence and ability to resist abuse and unwanted sexual experiences. In addition, it needs to build on the best available evidence as to what works in reducing teenage pregnancy and improving sexual health.

Sex and relationships education should support children now and in the future. It should help them move through puberty, into adolescence and through into adulthood confidently and with the skills and understanding they need to manage the physical, social and emotional changes that this involves. It needs to be mindful of children's early experiences and be based on their developmental and expressed needs. It should provide consistent messages, be continuous and progressive.

This process should support and enable young people to be aware of and enjoy their sexuality; develop positive values and a moral framework that will guide their decisions, judgements and behaviour; have confidence and self-esteem to value themselves and others; behave responsibly within sexual and personal relationships;

communicate effectively; have sufficient skills and information to protect themselves from unintended conceptions and sexually transmitted infections including HIV; neither exploit nor be exploited; and access confidential advice and support.

TAKING PARENTS SERIOUSLY: WHAT DO PARENTS WANT FROM SCHOOLS?

Despite an often strongly held belief that parents do not support sex and relationships education, the evidence suggests differently. Research shows that parents support sex and relationships education (National Foundation for Educational Research/ Health Education Authority, *Parents, Schools and Sex and Relationships Education*, 1994). Research by Walker has shown that they often feel ill equipped to talk to their children about sex and relationships ('A Qualitative Study of Parents' Experiences of Providing Sex and Relationships Education for their Children', *Health Education Journal* 60 (2), 2001). Many feel unable to do it because they feel embarrassed and/or lack the knowledge and skills about when and how to approach the subject. As a result they often look to schools to take on the job of talking to their children. Research also confirms that they would like their children to get more sex and relationships education than they do and at a younger age. They really want schools to take on some of the more 'difficult issues' such as abortion, sexuality and contraception.

THE EVIDENCE BASE FOR SEX AND RELATIONSHIPS EDUCATION

As noted before, the UK has one of the highest teenage pregnancy rates in Western Europe. Sexually transmitted infections including HIV continue to rise and we know that poor sexual health and early pregnancy is associated with poverty, disadvantage and low aspirations. If we look to our European neighbours, where teenage pregnancy rates are low and they have better sexual health morbidity than we do, it is clear that an open, honest approach to sex and relationships pays dividends. We have evidence of what constitutes effective sex and relationships education (see, for example, C. Meyrick and J. Swann, *An Overview of Effectiveness in Reducing Teenage Conceptions*, Health Education Authority, 1998) and this evidence base is the foundation on which to build effective sex and relationships education.

DEVELOPING EFFECTIVE SEX AND RELATIONSHIPS EDUCATION PROGRAMMES

Using the current evidence of effectiveness as a foundation, the following is a programme of what should be taught to children in schools. It incorporates an interpretation of the National Curriculum Science Order, the personal, social and health education and citizenship framework and the sex and relationships education guidance. The Sex Education Forum believes that this is a broad and balanced programme that should be an entitlement of all children and young people.

Key Stage 1 – ages 5 to 7
The science curriculum requires that pupils are able to recognize differences between themselves and others; to know and understand that humans and other animals can produce offspring and that their offspring grow into adults; and to know about the main external parts of the body. These biological aspects are only one part of sex and relationships education and the foundations of personal social development will be delivered through PSHE and citizenship.

By the end of Key Stage 1, pupils have learnt basic communication skills of listening and talking with others, can recognize and name a range of emotions, explain a range of feelings and ideas; recognize an unsafe situation; and talk with a trusted adult and ask for help.

They will also know and understand that babies need to be cared for and have thought about their responsibilities in caring for others.

Key Stage 2 – ages 7 to 11
The science curriculum requires that children know and understand the life processes common to humans and other animals including growth and reproduction and the main stages of the human lifecycle. Again, the personal and social development aspects of sex and relationships education and the explicit preparation for puberty and adolescence will be delivered through PSHE and citizenship.

By the end of Key Stage 2 pupils are able to listen to others, explain themselves, explore and discuss, describe and express emotions, recognize abuse and ask for help and manage the physical and emotional changes of puberty. They will know and understand: the physical and emotional changes of puberty; the range of relationships, including the importance of family and marriage, for the care and support of children; the effect of the media on forming attitudes; and infection and how safe routines can reduce the spread of viruses including HIV. Pupils will have had the opportunities to think about diversity and how it is important to listen to other opinions and respect differences.

Key Stage 3 – age 11 to 14
The science curriculum requires that pupils know and understand physical and emotional changes that take place during adolescence, human reproduction, including the menstrual cycle and fertilization and how the growth and reproduction of bacteria and the spread of viruses can affect health. To support them through adolescence sex and relationships education will be further developed through PSHE.

By the end of Key Stage 3 pupils will still continue to develop the whole range of personal and social skills needed for relationships with family and friends and to discuss relationships, recognize abuse and risk; resist unwanted pressure; recognize, express and manage emotions including loss caused by change, divorce and separation; and ask for help and seek advice from the appropriate services. They know and understand: how relationships affect well-being, and how family life including marriage supports the upbringing of children; about differences in relation to gender, sexuality and race and the impact of prejudice; about sexual health including contraception, STIs and HIV; how the media affects attitudes and public opinion; the law affecting sex and young people; and the significance of cultural and religious beliefs on all aspects of sexual health.

Key Stage 4 – age 14 to 16
The science curriculum requires that children and young people know and understand about hormonal control and the effect of sex hormones and how sex is determined in humans. Further preparation for adulthood will be delivered through PSHE and citizenship.

By the end of Key Stage 4 pupils have developed a confidence in their personal and social skills and are able to demonstrate assertive skills and an ability to discuss a range of moral, social and cultural issues such as age of consent, fertility treatment, abuse and exploitation, contraception and abortion. They also know and understand how contraception works and where to get advice, about STIs and HIV and safer sex; how risk taking affects sexual health and well-being; how alcohol and drug use can affect risk taking; the law affecting young people and sex; the range of advice and support in the local community and nationally. They will also have had opportunities to think about sexual identity, the consequence of sexual activity and relationships, values and how they affect behaviour and the benefit of stable relationships including marriage and family on parenting and bringing up children.

CONCLUSION

If teachers and others working in schools are to feel confident to teach children and young people about sex and relationships, we need to start discussing how we will deliver sex and relationships education that meets the needs of children and young people, addresses parents' concerns and meets the imperatives of public health and social health inequalities. This type of careful planning and discussion needs commitment. It will also mean sometimes agreeing to disagree and respecting the right of people to hold different beliefs.

If sex and relationships education continues to be dogged by moral and political rhetoric as well as polarized debates then – despite a well-developed evidence base and consensus on what constitutes good practice – children and young people will continue to be denied their entitlement to good-quality, effective sex and relationships education.

At the beginning of a new millennium, we have a choice in Britain. We can continue to believe that silence will ensure children and young people maintain their innocence and perpetuate a culture of worry, confusion and guilt when it comes to sex and relationships. Or we can use the evidence base and, as children and young people request, grasp the nettle. We can respond to their plea for better sex and relationships education that will help them to develop the knowledge, attitudes and skills to manage their relationships and sexual health effectively. Indeed, we cannot afford to do otherwise.

Essay Three

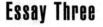

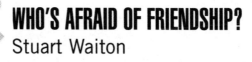

WHO'S AFRAID OF FRIENDSHIP?
Stuart Waiton

The debate surrounding the extension of sex education across the UK has been perceived as a battle between reformers who want a more open and relaxed attitude to sex and traditional moralists who think that sex education corrupts young minds and should be kept out of the classroom. Despite the image that this debate creates of open-minded liberals fighting off the bigots of the past, I argue in this essay that, with each new sexual health campaign and sex education initiative, teenagers' lives are becoming more and more regulated and controlled. In replacing the moral sermons of the past, government ministers and health promotion experts are developing a new framework for sex education. This sex education is based on the assumption that young people are in danger, not of committing acts of sin, but of being physically and emotionally damaged by sexual activity. Regardless of genuine attempts by some to adopt a more progressive and liberal approach to young people's lives, the outcome of this approach is that important rites of passage to adulthood are being undermined by concerned adults, worried about the potentially risky and abusive relationships that teenagers are having with one another.

THE DANGERS OF SEX 'TOO EARLY'

Within the literature on both teenage pregnancies and sex education, despite the call for a more open and honest dialogue about sex, the need for teenagers to 'delay having sex' is considered paramount. Tony Blair, in his introduction to the Social Exclusion Unit (SEU) report on teenage pregnancy, states: 'I don't believe young people should have sex before they are 16.' This is not simply a personal message from a Christian prime minister, but is a view that is endorsed and reiterated by almost every document on the subject of teenage sex. The *Sex and Relationships Education Guidance* from the Department for Education and Employment (DfEE) (2000), for example, explains that the key task for schools is to reduce teenage pregnancies by giving advice on contraception and on 'delaying sexual activity'.

Both the guidance document and the SEU report stress the importance of empowering young people, via assertiveness training and improving their knowledge of sex and relationships, so that they can avoid having sex 'too early'. The ex-health minister Tessa Jowell in an article in the *Independent*, described an 'amazing project' she visited in the Bronx, New York, which 'warned the pupils against being browbeaten by their peers into having sex too young', by them 'learning to say "no" or "not yet".' But how is the concern about having sex 'too early' justified? Do the arguments made in favour of delaying sex make sense?

GOVERNMENT WARNING: SEX CAN SERIOUSLY DAMAGE YOUR HEALTH

One argument for delaying sex contends that sex constitutes a risk to health. In order to avoid this risk, it is argued, sex education needs to take an 'open and honest' approach and provide young people with the 'facts' about sex. This sounds reasonable, but the problem with this openness, honesty and delivery of facts, is that the emphasis is almost invariably placed on providing information that exaggerates the health risks of sexual activity.

The case of HIV/AIDS awareness (something that schools *must* teach) is the most blatant example of how today's 'non judgmental', objective and scientific approach to sex education is anything but scientific. Despite reports in the 1980s and 90s about the coming AIDS epidemic, by 1999, outside of high-risk groups, only 171 people had contracted the AIDS virus via heterosexual sex (M. Fitzpatrick, *The Tyranny of Health*, 2000). This fact is, however, not part of the sex 'education' that young people receive today. Despite the low risk of contracting HIV, 'AIDS awareness' must, according to the law, be taught to children.

The latest 'epidemic' promoted by sexual health educators is chlamydia. Chlamydia hit the headlines in England in 1999, with talk of an 'invisible bug leaving women infertile'. Up to 100,000 women, it was claimed, could find themselves unable to have children within the next decade. A columnist in the *Daily Mail* explained that: 'Nature has ways of making us see sense and in the same way that AIDS was a warning to gays to amend their promiscuous ways, the sexually transmitted disease chlamydia is now warning girls to keep their virginity firmly intact.' This predictable warning from a newspaper notorious for stoking up fears about teenage sex has been more than matched by 'information' provided by liberal sex educators.

A leaflet campaign about chlamydia in England and Wales, while flagging up the dangers of this disease that has few symptoms and can make a woman infertile, failed to mention the fact that it is extremely easy to treat with a simple course of antibiotics. This, to its credit, is something the Health Education Board for Scotland's (HEBS) leaflet on the subject does point out. However, the justification for all the concern about the increase in this disease is debatable. Headlines which have stated that the diagnosis of chlamydia 'that can lead to infertility' has increased by 75 per cent over the last five years need to be examined.

First, that the diagnosis of the infection has increased does not mean the number of people catching it has increased. The incidence of chlamydia up to 1990, for example, was hidden within figures for non-specific urethritis because it was difficult to detect. Today medical advances mean chlamydia can be identified more easily and so figures have increased over the last ten years. Also, the increase in the number of cases diagnosed is gained from people who visit clinics and, therefore, give no indication of the level of infection of the general population. An increase in the number of young people visiting clinics is likely to increase the rate of detection of a disease and, as the *Healthy Respect* pamphlet published by Lothian Health Authority points out, 'recent figures indicate a dramatic increase in the number of 16–24 year olds attending genito-urinary medicine clinics.' More check-ups mean the figures for the infection increase, but does not mean the incidence itself has increased, simply that more people have been diagnosed as having chlamydia.

Finally, the talk of chlamydia 'leading to infertility', is more confusing than clarifying. According to a Glasgow-based specialist in sexually transmitted infections, the chances of becoming infertile from catching chlamydia are about 100 to one. The focus on, and discovery of, an increase in the diagnosis of chlamydia appears to have more to do with new medical practices backed up with a greater interest by the professionals in the 'sexual health' of young people rather than an increase in the rate of infection.

A convincing explanation for the 'rise of chlamydia' is therefore less straightforward than it has been presented to be. But the high level of concern about infertility has an important outcome, in that it creates an unnecessary level of anxiety for young women. Infertility is the extreme rather than the norm. The condition has always existed, simply under another name and infertility rates may not be noticeably increasing. The value of promoting high-profile warnings about chlamydia is dubious indeed. In sum, 'information' about the health risks of sex appears to constitute more a modern-day version of the warning 'nature has ways of making us see sense', than an objective assessment of the likelihood of teenagers contracting sexually transmitted diseases and suffering serious health problems from them.

THE TEENAGE PREGNANCY 'PROBLEM'

Another vehicle for promoting the problem of sex 'too early' is the issue of teenage pregnancy. The 'problem' of teenage pregnancy has, over the last few years, become central to the drive for more and better sex education. An issue, which was originally politicized by Conservative politicians in their attack on 'underclass scroungers', has now been adopted as a central element in New Labour's strategy to combat 'social exclusion'. Interestingly, despite the reality that most teenage pregnancies and teenage mothers are found within economically poor areas, the 'problem' of teenage pregnancies has been used by Tony Blair to justify more sex education for all – including those young people living in 'leafy suburbs.'

It is worth noting, amid tabloid tales of 12-year-olds getting pregnant, that while concern about this issue has rocketed, the number of teenagers getting pregnant has not. In Scotland, for example, the number getting pregnant has gradually declined over recent years. Also in England, while 90,000 teenagers became pregnant in 1997 (a figure that is often used to highlight the big 'social problem' of 'teen sex') only 7,700 conceptions were to under 16-year-olds (the vast majority of these being to 15-year-olds) of which 3,700 resulted in births. Despite these relatively small numbers, however, the 'problems' of teenage pregnancy and teenage motherhood, have been used to justify more sex education for all young people in the UK.

In this discussion about teenage pregnancies, an issue of concern is that young people are far more 'sexual' and sexually active than ever before and a perception has been cultivated that 'if something isn't done' the age of young people having sex will continue to get ever lower. However, while the average age of first-time sex is currently 17, 40 years ago it was between 20 and 21. In other words it has taken 40 years for the age of first-time sex to fall by between three and four years. But even this figure does not tell the whole story of the changing age of first sex. Despite the concern raised by the SEU report that 'the number of young people sexually active by the age of 16' has 'doubled between 1965 and 1991', backed up by headlines such as 'Children of eight are now reaching puberty, and pre-teen sex in not unusual' (*The Observer*, 18 June 2000), this is not a linear trend set to continue. Indeed, the research this 'doubling' refers to actually shows that for boys, the increase in 'young people sexually active by the age of 16', came between 1965 and 1975 and from then until 1991 there was almost no increase. For girls, there appears to be a more gradual increase over time, which has led to approximately one third of school-age teenagers saying they are sexually active. However, this greater equalization of the age of first sex between boys and girls should be interpreted as a positive reflection of women's growing equality rather than a political, social and moral problem.

The justifications discussed so far, for problematizing sex 'too early', make little sense. Sex is not a significant risk to the health of teenagers and neither is teenage pregnancy the major social problem it is presented to be. In the sections that follow, I will argue that warnings about the dangers of sex are not only baseless, they actually do more harm than good.

CONTRACEPTION AND MIXED MESSAGES

The issue of contraception has inevitably come to the fore, as the 'problem' of teenage pregnancy has risen up the political agenda. It is certainly the case that young people need easy-access contraception. But the desire to prevent young people from having sex 'too early' means that discussion of contraception is dogged by confusing signals, which make contraceptive use less likely.

The Netherlands is often held up as a good example of the impact that sex education has on reducing the level of unwanted pregnancies. However, it is not the message to delay having sex that has made the difference, but the far greater and more effective use of contraceptives. The proportion of young people using contraception at first intercourse is 85 per cent, compared with 50 per cent in the UK. But young people in the Netherlands are not – after receiving sex education lessons – having sex any later than young people in the UK. However, crucially, in the Netherlands, sex among teenagers is not seen as a problem and something to be avoided – which means that for young women in particular, the more relaxed atmosphere surrounding sex makes it easier for them to go on the pill.

This approach is a far cry from the mixed messages young people receive in Britain. Growing concern about teenage mothers in the UK means there is a constant pressure regarding contraception, to make it more readily available. However, the Government is still uncomfortable with confidently promoting the pill or morning-after pill, largely because this would not sit well with the message that young people should avoid having sex if possible. The promotion of condoms – a less effective form of contraception than the pill – is, however, widespread. This is, first, because it endorses the Government's preoccupation with making young men 'more responsible' for their sex lives and second, because condoms are bound up with the issue of disease and safety.

Given this confused approach by the Government, it is disingenuous in the extreme to imagine that young people will find it easy to ask for contraception. As long as they live in a society that stigmatizes sex as diseased, irresponsible and dangerous, the rates of contraceptive use achieved in the Netherlands are likely to remain unattainable.

WHO NEEDS RELATIONSHIPS EDUCATION?

Perhaps the most damaging aspect of sex education today is the increasing emphasis on relationships education. This concept is now at the heart of sex education with sex education itself becoming an increasingly prominent part of personal social and health education (PSHE). PSHE in its turn is becoming more central to the national curriculum, with each curriculum subject (English, history, science and so on) contributing to the PSHE agenda, which will have its own code of practice and targets monitored by OFSTED. This development is helping to transform sex and relationship education from being a 'cor!' subject into a core subject. In the past it was the adult world and particularly the world of education that usefully would take young people's minds off sex and relationships and get them to think about issues broader than their own personal lives. Today, however, the obsession with personal problems is being promoted within schools not only though sex and relationships education but throughout PSHE and even within the general curriculum.

Of course, sex and relationships education is not education at all. It is not based on an academic discipline to help develop abstract thinking like English or maths. Neither does it develop educational 'skills' like art or craft and design. In English, for example, students can discuss jealousy or love through characters in a book, from a distance and within a context. Sex and relationships education, in comparison, is more like religious instruction. It is not about taking a distance from the subject and developing critical thinking, it is about trying to imbue young people with a set of values. In sex education classes, students do not discuss AIDS as an 'issue' or a matter for debate, but as a disease they must be 'aware' of. Young people in the class may raise questions, but the point of 'education' about AIDS is purely to 'raise awareness'. Indeed, if teenagers were leaving their sex education classes thinking that AIDS was not a problem, that chlamydia had been hyped out of all proportion and that sex was a purely recreational, rather than a 'responsible' activity, the teacher of this class would no doubt be under investigation from OFSTED inspectors.

Despite all the talk about making sex education more open and honest, the reverse looks set to develop. Structured within the curriculum, with set packs and guidelines being developed about what should and should not be taught, the scope for flexibility and 'the personal touch' is actually reduced. When 'relationships' were not part of 'education' as such, and the guidelines for what can and cannot be discussed were far less prescriptive, there was always scope for a teacher to give advice to a pupil – more as a friend than as a teacher. Today, however, in the *Sex and Relationship Education Guidance* notes, it is explained that teachers must 'ensure that pupils know that teachers cannot offer unconditional confidentiality.' The more legalistic arrangement between teacher and pupil established here means that the relationship between two human beings is contractualized and any teacher giving confidential advice in the future could face disciplinary measures.

This is bad enough but perhaps worse still is the patronizing assumption, at the centre of the rationale for relationship education, that young people are all vulnerable – not just physically but also emotionally – and in need of support. Girls, traditionally portrayed as the 'weaker sex', are now depicted as being pushed into having sex by both media images (teenagers apparently believe everything they watch on TV) and by boys. As an article in *The Scotsman* explained, of the Government's latest sex education campaign: 'The campaign is designed to combat peer pressure which experts believe is forcing girls as young as 11 and 12 into having sex.' The traditional conservative image of the sexless, fragile girl needing support to defend her honour from lustful boys is replicated here through the prism of the vulnerable teenager.

The answer, it is argued, is to help young women through assertiveness training to develop their self-esteem, thus empowering them to say 'no' to sex. That an assertive girl may use her training and newly discovered self-esteem to get into her boyfriend's jeans, is never considered. Neither is the possibility that a young woman may gain self-esteem, rather than lose it, by having sex.

Significantly, the key difference with today's image of boys and girls from the past, is that now boys are also seen as being vulnerable and in need of support. Indeed, teenage boys have become the main focus of relationship education, because it is believed their vulnerabilities, unlike those of 'emotional' girls, are hidden behind a macho mask. The extreme example of 'rising male suicide rates', allegedly caused by 'masculine values' acting as a barrier to asking for help, is given as a key reason to develop further intervention in the sex lives of young boys.

While girls are pressurized by boys, boys, it is argued, also face peer pressure to 'act like a man' and have sex 'too early'. Peer pressure, in the SEU report on teenage pregnancy, is described as a 'general problem'. The Sex Education Forum (SEF) believes this problem results in a lack of 'empathetic interpersonal problem solving by virtue of the tendency of boys to play in groups.' Because boys play in groups, it is argued, 'males (consciously or otherwise) exclude themselves or are excluded from the warmth of human relations.' Gill Lenderyou, of the SEF, argues in the pamphlet *Let's hear it for the boys!* that: '... because boys hang about in groups there are limited opportunities for talking about feelings, emotions and fears.' 'It all feels a bit grim,' she explains, 'growing up as a boy, alone and alienated and relying on the peer group which also fosters that aloneness.'

As an ex-boy myself, and one that grew up with a peer group of 'lads', I do not recognize this picture. The caricature of girls as pressured into sex, presented by the SEF, is here matched by an equally caricatured view of boys, who, while vulnerable underneath are en masse unable to express their emotions to one another without the support of a teacher or counsellor.

The flipside of the image of the teenage boy as vulnerable is the creation of the 'abusive lad'. In *Let's hear it for the boys!* there is a palpable distaste for the boys who a few pages earlier were described as being so vulnerable. Indeed, the authors appear to be trying to convince themselves that these villainous boys are worth saving: 'We need to examine our own negative perceptions and expectations of boys,' they warn. 'As workers,' they explain, 'we need to maintain our liking for boys while challenging their sometimes sexist and homophobic opinions.' In Chapter 2, educational consultant Graham Wild writes, 'We need to separate our dislike of the boys' behaviour from them as people.' Boys, while victims of peer pressure themselves, are also presented here as all-round bullies and sexist homophobes. Without the intervention of liberal-minded professionals, with their relationship education pack in hand, these 'vulnerable' boys, it is assumed, will be locked behind their macho and potentially abusive mask.

It is worth pointing out here that the use of 'sexist', caricatured images and language used by boys is often a reflection of their immaturity and their attempt to develop a sense of themselves as boys. To perceive young boys who use 'sexist' language, as the male chauvinists of the future is not only premature but wrong. As these boys grow up and develop relationships beyond their peer groups they also grow out of this behaviour as it becomes increasingly inapporiate for most of the social circumstances in which they find themselves. The sexist men of the future will emerge out of many individual and social experiences but cannot be identified in the 'boy talk' of children or adolescents.

The discussion about peer pressure within young people's sexual relationships and the perception of relationships between teenage boys and girls as potentially abusive, has some dangerous and authoritarian consequences. The latest NSPCC research on sexual abuse of children, for example, argued that the main sexual abusers of children were other children – specifically those people who 'call themselves boyfriend and girlfriend'. A piece of research by the Zero Tolerance group in Scotland, claimed to have uncovered the shocking fact that most young people believe 'forced sex' is acceptable. The only way this presentation of young people as would-be or actual rapists and abusers can be explained is if the sexual fumbling of teenagers is seen through the eyes and laws of adult relationships. In the minds of the NSPCC and Zero Tolerance 'trying it on' has become the same thing as sexual abuse. The unfortunate and inevitable result of this perception of young people, as abusers and victims of abuse, is that the law steps in and children as young as ten start to be placed on the sexual offenders register for little more than playing doctors and nurses.

◈ ● ●
● ● CONCLUSION: WHY YOUNG PEOPLE'S
● ● ◈ PEERS ARE NOT THEIR ENEMIES

Through the establishment of relationship education in schools, an area of young people's lives, which up until recently was left alone, has become both professionalized and problematized. And rather than allowing young people to develop their own network of friends to discuss sex and relationships, an attempt is being made to break the 'power' of the peer group, and in its place establish a network of teachers, counsellors and health specialists. By replacing peers with professionals, the incredibly important framework that peer groups and friendships provide for young people's development will potentially be undermined.

The idea expressed in *Let's hear it for the boys!*, that boys only ever hang around in groups and are therefore unable to discuss emotional issues, is clearly not true. While they do hang about in groups, as do some girls, invariably they also have close individual friendships within these groups. Indeed in terms of boys' ability or inability to express emotions to friends, a review of research on peer relations found that, while 'males are less likely to engage in intimate disclosure (than girls), 40 per cent of the close male friendships studied did involve a high degree of mutual intimacy' (W. A. Corsaro and Donna Eder, 'Children's Peer Culture', *Annual Review of Sociology*, 1990). In fact, individual differences of children appear to be as important as gender differences when looking at whether or not they have intimate relationships.

It is also a mistake to see peer groups as restricting teenagers' emotional development and understanding of sex and relationships. It is worth noting that, while many young people do cite peer pressure as a factor in why they first had sex when they did, they are generally expressing experience not of an abusive relationship but the fact that they were growing up. In *Education in Sex and Personal Relationships* (Isobel Allen, Policy Studies Institute, 1987) it was found that peer pressure to have sex was felt much more by 16-year-olds than 14-year-olds. This was not because they were being bullied but because more friends at this age are either having sex or thinking about having sex.

Peer groups are vital to young people because they act as a crutch for individuals who do not fully understand themselves or the adult world they live in. By developing a level of trust and intimacy they provide a forum in which ideas can be tried out. This is often done in the third person or through gossip and 'mickey taking', but through this process, a greater awareness of issues and concerns is explored. Child psychologists Parker and Gottman, in the *Annual Review of Sociology*, noted that while gossip was primarily used for group solidarity in early adolescence, 'in later adolescence, gossip provided an entry into the psychological exploration of the self.'

Young people use 'the group' environment to develop themselves as individuals in their move towards independence and adulthood. The process whereby children and young people stop looking to adults for personal guidance is an important one. In the way that children stop 'telling tales to teacher' as they get older, young people need to learn how to think about, and resolve, their own personal problems rather than relying on an adult to always be there for them. This development is crucial if teenagers are to start taking personal responsibility for themselves. Unfortunately, the development of relationship education runs the risk of undermining this process by encouraging young people to resolve their personal problems through the relationship 'expert'.

Young people may need some facts from adults, but when discussing intimate matters they should be left alone. At different ages, some young people will not fully understand aspects of love, death and relationships, but as they mature – with the help of their friends – this develops and, equally important, so too does the intimate network of friendships.

Professional intervention into young people's personal lives has a number of dangers. For example, the promotion of the 'correct relationship' within relationship education, as the 'stable loving relationship', will be entirely inappropriate for many young people. As the American sociologist Rosalind Petchesky explains, 'Sporadic risk taking or exploratory formats of sexual behaviour may be endemic to early adolescence', with adult forms of behaviour such as 'going steady, being potentially futile or destructive' (*Abortion and Woman's Choice*, 1990). Also, the trend to see teenagers' sexual relationships as abusive, confuses the type of immature, unsure, experimental relationships that teenagers are having. The feminist idea of 'no means no' in the context of adolescent relationships, where many of the steps to full sex take young people into unknown territory and break down barriers, is entirely inappropriate and is likely simply to confuse young people further.

While an understanding of human reproduction is an important element of education, the rest of the 'awareness' raising surrounding sex and relationship education is not. The formalization, the professionalization and indeed the politicization of sex, and particularly of relationships, looks set to undermine rather than assist the development of intimate relationships among teenagers.

Essay Four

THE FAILURE OF SEX EDUCATION
Peter Hitchens

It is very hard to be innocent in modern Britain. Advertising on television, on posters and on the radio, is drenched in sexual innuendo. Television programmes rely almost entirely on sex and violence to raise their drooping audience figures. The playgrounds of primary schools echo with sexual taunts and jibes. Rock music, which is now almost compulsory in the lives of even the youngest, is full of sexual expression and desire. And then there is sex education, the details of which we shall come to a little later, with its condoms, bananas, diagrams and exercises to break down inhibition. And inhibition most certainly is broken down, as all can see in a world in which 14-year-old boys impregnate 12-year-old girls and are proud of it, and primary school pupils are charged with rape. Yet, amid all this, we are expected to believe that somewhere out there, there are still significant numbers of young people who do not know how babies are made and for whom the connection between intercourse and pregnancy, or intercourse and certain diseases, is a mystery.

As recently as July 2001 *Doctor* magazine produced a survey claiming that some young people believe that, if you close your eyes, stand on a phone book or drink milk during sex you will not get pregnant. One pro-sex education pressure group responded to this by saying: 'Too often young people tell us that the information they are given about sex is too little, too late and that it is too biological. They need plain speaking and impartial information.' Whatever does this mean? What could be more plain spoken and impartial than biology, with its cool, unemotional diagrams of this inserted into that, this swimming there and colliding with that and the subsequent development of a new person who, short of bloody violence, cannot then be prevented from arriving in the world by the traditional method?

Perhaps in some yearning fashion, the half-formed, lonely and morally illiterate children who go off and make babies have responded rationally to the impartiality of what has been shown to them. They have perhaps been moved by the simple beauty of it and its clear purpose – and in a world lacking both beauty and purpose they may have sought those things. If they needed plain speaking, it was of the kind that is now practically outlawed in the schools, plain speaking about right and wrong, about actions having consequences, about responsibility and maturity, obligation and morality. A baby is a lovely thing, but it demands a heavy price in the hard, old-fashioned currency of duty. What is more, that price must be paid in full and without delay, with no interest free credit allowed and no post-dated cheque. No amount of counselling or social security or other intervention can make up for parental commitment if it is absent.

But that, I suppose, is another issue. The real question before us is actually much simpler. How is it that the arguments used in favour of sex education are so transparently ridiculous, yet nobody seems to notice or care? The human race managed to reproduce for thousands of years before there was education of any kind, let alone sex education. Why, in the twentieth and twenty-first centuries, were we suddenly plunged into this black night of ignorance so great that pedagogues must be trained to wave condoms about in the classroom and use rude words in front of seven-year-olds? And, if education is such an effective way of banishing ignorance from the land, why is it that the more of this sex instruction there is the more unwanted irresponsible pregnancies and sexually transmitted diseases there are? Surely, the main message of the last half-century is that sex education has failed in its supposed purpose. In which case it is worth asking if this is its true purpose at all.

◇ ● ●
● ●
● ● ◇ **SEX EDUCATION: A BRIEF HISTORY**

None of this controversy is even slightly new, although it is interesting that in each generation it has taken a slightly, but significantly different shape. Agitation for sex education in schools was already growing in the 1930s, especially in the 'advanced' and 'progressive' Socialist authorities such as the London County Council. In September 1935 the *News Chronicle* reported that the LCC education committee:

> ... has been considering the need for equipping boys and girls in the residential schools, who are nearing the age at which they leave school, with such knowledge of sex questions as would enable them to approach these matters in a clean and proper state of mind when they start working life.

But, significantly, this 'equipping' was restricted to the children in 'residential schools', who were not living at home, and could not be expected to have learned about these things from their parents. The LCC had a formal ban on sex education throughout its ordinary schools which had been in force since 1914, a ban that would not in the end be lifted until February 1949. 'Sex,' the council then decided in those newly progressive times, 'should be introduced into as many lessons – such as hygiene and biology – as possible.' However, it was careful to placate worried parents and clergymen by making clear that it would remain biological and dispassionate. There should not, it ruled firmly, 'be special lessons on sex instruction.'

The issue first became politically important during World War II, lifted into prominence by the excuse that wartime sexual mores had exposed the new generation to far greater risks of venereal disease than ever before. This was the justification given in November 1943 when the Board of Education issued a pamphlet urging local authorities in England and Wales to offer courses on sex education not to children, but to teachers and youth leaders, to equip them to 'open up the subject'. An 'official survey' was said to have shown that 'far too many children have little balanced knowledge of sex.' But this was to be so no longer: 'The proverbial gooseberry bush, the stork or the doctor's bag may, it is hoped, now be finally discarded.' Almost 58 years later, the gooseberry bush seems merely to have given way to the telephone directory, the eyes-shut method or the glass of milk. But did anyone ever really believe in the gooseberry bush or the stork? And do they now believe in the efficacy of jumping up and down afterwards as a method of post-coital contraception?

Let us march forward, as everyone was doing in those days, to February 1949, when the *Sunday Pictorial*, forerunner of today's *Sunday Mirror*, dealt with, yes, 'a question of vital importance to every parent in Britain – WHO SHOULD BE RESPONSIBLE [their emphasis] FOR THE SEX EDUCATION OF OUR CHILDREN -THE PARENTS OR THE SCHOOL AUTHORITIES?' Beneath a winsome photograph of a little girl cuddling a foal, the *Sunday Pictorial* made its own view clear, praising those enlightened authorities who had even then 'faced the problem frankly'.

Drawing attention to its own recent series of articles on the birth of a baby, the paper complained that 'the duty of imparting sex knowledge has hitherto fallen ONLY on their parents. Unfortunately, this duty has been neglected only too often... Too many children – of this generation and of those past – have acquired sex knowledge in a furtive and underhand manner. They have half-learned the truth through sniggering innuendo, brash experimentation and smutty jokes.' Little did its editors know that this method of sex education would, half a century later, become the main source material of television light entertainment. Neither, perhaps, did they suspect that their sweetly innocent campaign might have helped to create a world in which smut emerged from behind the bikesheds and became seriously big business.

Yet again, one of the openly stated purposes of sex education has not merely not been achieved, but has been actively subverted since sex education became common. Was there ever a smuttier time than this, the start of the twenty-first century? Were dirty jokes and dirty minds ever so widespread as they are now? We used to be told that smut was simply a response to puritanism. But as puritanism has disappeared from the world, smut has become a legitimate route to riches and status in society. But, there, I am disgressing again into matters which are allegedly irrelevant to the subject.

The really striking difference between the sex education campaigners of the past and those of today is the cautious modesty of the *Sunday Pictorial*'s ideas on what should constitute sex education. In the junior schools it says 'the keeping of pets would provoke further questions and nature study lessons would provide some opportunities for a more direct approach... In secondary schools it might be possible to include in the first year of a general science course a simple outline of physiology, including reproduction.'

The newspaper's intervention followed a now forgotten quarrel in the town of Maltby in Yorkshire, where parents petitioned against 'facts of life' talks in the local secondary modern girls' school. Mrs Jessie Tallantire, wife of the local cinema manager, said she thought it was:

> ... scandalous that such a subject should be put over by full blackboard drawings. The things our daughters know now at the age of 11 horrify us. My daughter attended sex lectures last week and on Friday the lecture took up a double period – yet she did not have one arithmetic lesson all the week... I think arithmetic should come first.

Her complaint was prophetic. Half a century later children were emerging from school after 11 years unable to multiply seven by nine, but quite capable of multiplying themselves.

The response of the West Riding education authority, as it then was, was to brief reporters that the lectures aimed to 'sweep away the mystery of sex for adolescents and make them see it was something to be accepted naturally and casually and not whispered about in corners.' Not all authorities took the same view. The following year Edinburgh's deputy director of education told sixth-formers in the Scottish capital that: 'Sex teaching is primarily a job for the home. In a matter as important as this parents should take the responsibility themselves.' Imagine what would happen to any education bureaucrat who dared to suggest this now.

By 1950 there were complaints from rural Wiltshire that immorality among children might have resulted from the sex lessons they had been given. A boy and girl aged 12 and 11 were alleged to have been found 'to have practised what had been taught in school sex lectures.' Interestingly, the authorities denied that they had ever taught what was then called 'birth control', which was then still very much taboo and restricted to those who were married.

By 1960 a church survey in south London showed 'an alarming ignorance, misunderstanding and departure from tradition in the sexual code of young people', although it was not clear if this was because they had too much sex instruction or too little. By 1963 the story had now slipped into the familiar modern pattern as it was disclosed that 'more sex education is to be given in Norwich schools to curb a rise in the number of unmarried mothers.' It was announced that the illegitimacy rate had reached 7.7 per cent, compared with 5.9 per cent nationally. Fourteen of the unmarried mothers in Norwich were aged 16 and under – four of them schoolgirls. The chairman of the Norwich education committee complained 'I'm surprised the figures are not higher in view of the conditions in which young people live today. On TV, radio and in the national press there is a general lowering, not only of morals but of truth.' It is sad to think what he and his committee would make of the programme *Big Brother*, where a slack-jawed nation watched to see if two near-strangers might have sex with each other in front of network TV cameras. As for the present rate of illegitimacy, nearly 40 per cent, words would probably fail them.

THE FAILURE OF SEX EDUCATION

Yet words need not fail us, if we will only keep hold of sense and logic. The years since the people of Norwich quite rightly panicked at an illegitimacy rate of 7.7 per cent have been a powerful disproof of the sex educators' arguments. Children are now taught incomparably more about sex, directly and without inhibition, than they were ever taught then. They can go to doctors and ask for contraceptive advice in the knowledge that their parents will not be told about it. They can see more or less explicit posters advertising condoms on bus shelters and highly explicit machines selling them in public lavatories, so that most of them have both the money and the knowledge to get hold of these things without the puce-faced embarrassment which faced earlier generations. In many parts of the country they can buy 'morning-after pills' with few restrictions and in some places they can get them for nothing, although nobody will tell them that the idea of post-coital emergency contraception was originally developed by a vet trying to prevent a pedigree bitch from becoming pregnant by a wayward mongrel.

If it were possible to make it easier for young people to have uninhibited yet sterile sex, then the social workers, the sex educators and their government allies would undoubtedly spend the money to do so and even more money to publicize what they had done. It may well be that the morning-after pill, if it is given away freely enough, will finally do what no other sex education initiative has done and bring down the illegitimacy rate. But it will do so only by destroying unborn lives in unprecedented numbers. I choose my words carefully. Whether you believe that unborn life is the same as life or whether you believe that the morning after pill is in effect an abortion pill, it is unarguable that lives, which would otherwise have taken place, will be snuffed out by it.

Many will continue to think that this is preferable to the old way, in which illegitimacy was either prevented by moral barriers, censure, stigma and shame, or cancelled by marriage. And there we really have it. From the start, sex education has been the chosen tool of those who wished to liberate sex from shame, in the belief that by doing so they would liberate the masses from a monstrous repression. They have seen sexual liberation as equivalent to political and economic liberation and have viewed sexual taboos as an instrument of reactionary authority.

This is the reason for the power and influence of the sex education lobby, despite its blatant failure and despite the oddness of the whole idea. Most of us are naturally suspicious of people who want to talk to other people's children about sex. We see it as at best peculiar and at worst as creepy and alarming. Most parents do not much want to tell their own children about sex and dread the first questions on the subject. Somehow the organizations which have campaigned for the right of officials and teachers and doctors positively to pester the young about the subject have won respectability and more, than respectability, a kind of admiration for their courage. Yet their excuses have been so thin. Venereal disease was a wartime problem, not because of ignorance, but because of the corrosive effect of modern war on families and marriage and also on restraint. The mass conscription of able-bodied young men, their disappearance into danger for months, years and sometimes forever, placed an impossible strain on many marriages and weakened the authority of parents over their children. The arrival of huge numbers of young, unattached and comparatively wealthy American servicemen, just at the moment when husbands and fathers were away fighting, led inevitably to promiscuity and licence.

Add to that the confusion, fatalism and destruction of the familiar brought about by air raids, direction of labour and evacuation and only a nation of saints could have coped without a great increase in illegitimacy, adultery, fornication and venereal disease. It is self-evidently ridiculous to suggest that better sex education could have made any important difference. It could, at best, have slightly mitigated the effects. You might as well issue umbrellas to people in the path of a hurricane. What actually helped in the end was the temporary restoration of morality and marriage which took place in the years after the war.

We know now that the contraceptive pill – which would transform the whole significance of sex in the 1960s – was not a value-neutral result of impartial scientific enquiry. It was developed largely at the prompting of the radical sexual liberationist, Margaret Sanger. The programme of experiments for the pill was made possible by cash help from Katharine Dexter McCormick, an eccentric millionairess, who believed motherhood was a form of tyranny. Sex education also has political and ethical baggage. Its pioneers in Britain seem to have come mainly from the political left, especially local government power bases of 'progressive' thinking such as the London County Council. Their influence over local government, with its responsibility for schools, gave them the chance to put their ideas into practice long before what is now known as political correctness had penetrated the central government machine and the top levels of the political parties.

INCREASING STATE POWER AND UNDERMINING THE FAMILY AND PARENTS

My own explanation for the dedication of these campaigners and for their political affiliations is that there is an inherent conflict between the married family and the modern state, which by making itself the benevolent all-encompassing source of learning, training, guidance, welfare and security must constantly increase its powers at the expense of parents. Lady Helen Brook, founder of the Brook Advisory Centres set up to give contraceptive advice to the unmarried (in the days when the distinction still mattered), wrote to *The Times* on 16 February 1980: 'From birth to death it is now the privilege of the parental state to take major decisions – objective, unemotional, the state weighs up what is best for the child.' In the years that followed, the 'family planning' lobby achieved a number of legal changes which destroyed parental authority over contraceptive advice and over the distribution of contraceptives, so ensuring that the morality of home and family were weakened and undermined and replaced by the amorality of the state.

As for sex education itself, it long ago ceased to be confined to biological description or even physical instruction and demonstration. In a survey of local authority sex education policies for the Family Education Trust, Paul Atkin recorded that: 'All sex education guides studied were implicitly hostile to the view that the two-parent family based on marriage was the best possible place for children to grow and develop. Writers of many local education authority syllabuses go to imaginative and often ridiculous lengths to avoid references to traditional family life.' Schools now also deal with this area of morality and culture in the growing fields of personal, health and social instruction, and the planned introduction of 'citizenship education' into the national curriculum.

In the summer of 2001 this process was taken a stage further. The Government set up a General Teaching Council for England (similar bodies exist in Wales and Scotland, although their developments and rules are not identical). Teachers cannot be employed in the state sector in England unless they are members of this body. The GTC has issued a draft code of practice which, if approved, will have a powerful effect on sex education. Its Clause 5 states that: 'Teachers recognise diversity, and work to ensure the rights of individuals to develop. They fully respect differences of gender, marital status, religion, colour, race, ethnicity, sexual orientation and disability. Teacher professionalism involves challenging prejudice and stereotypes to ensure equality of opportunity.' By equating 'sexual orientation' and marital status' with race, this clause classifies traditional Christian teaching on marriage and homosexual acts as being equivalent to racial prejudice.

If this clause is included in the final code, still under discussion in January 2002, it is bound to affect any future disciplinary hearings, not to mention recruitment of new teachers and promotion of existing ones. It would greatly limit the teacher's freedom of speech in class discussions on these issues and make a robust defence of the Christian married family impossible. Other teachers or pupils could claim that they had been offended or insulted by discrimination against their 'orientation'. Local authority workers who wished to preach homosexual equality and were refused access to classes by teachers who disapproved could complain, as could parents. The resulting cases, if they reached employment tribunals, could not fail to be affected by the existence of this clause.

CONCLUSION

I think it is fair to see sex education as just one part of a far wider campaign, rooted in the social radicalism of the early twentieth century, against traditional morality and the traditional family. Radicals have for many years seen both these as powerful conservative forces opposed to the march of 'progress' and it is hardly surprising that they have sought to undermine them. What is surprising is that they have come up against so little resistance so far. Perhaps this is because the era in which the family weakened and the state increased its powers has also been one either of wars, in which all could believe they were serving a high common purpose, or ever-increasing prosperity, when the delusion of permanent progress towards a perfect society could be maintained.

As prosperity falters, and the moral consequences of the death of marriage become apparent, the time has come for those who have doubts about sex education and the immoral teaching of the state in general to speak out. If there is a pendulum, it has swung too far. It may well be that our ancestors were too prudish, their morality too narrow and unforgiving, too inclined to punish the innocent along with the guilty and too harsh in their sanctions.

But in an age when millions of people watch a television series in the hope that they will see two people take part in the sex act, live on screen, a hope which was disappointed this year but will doubtless be fulfilled before long; when small children know the full vocabulary of sexual coarseness; when modesty and privacy have practically disappeared from the lives of millions; when so many children are growing up bereft of a proper family life, of the necessary examples of steadfastness, constancy and responsibility without which they will have to struggle with all their might to be decent human beings and will often fail; in such an age it is reasonable to ask if we might reconsider what we have done.

Those who have pursued change and reform in the name of progress, civilization and compassion must surely now be wondering if what they did was right. We who disagree with them should be merciful to them. The ugly facts are now all on our side. We do not need to gloat and we should not rub their noses in the disastrous statistics of abortions, illegitimate births, one-parent families, divorce, rape, sexual diseases and the rest. For the important thing is to change these facts for the better and, therefore, if it is at all possible, all decent people should be allies against the disaster that has overtaken family life in this country.

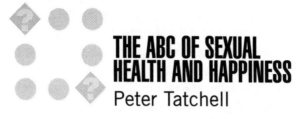

THE ABC OF SEXUAL HEALTH AND HAPPINESS
Peter Tatchell

Sex and love are two of the most important things in our lives. They can, and should, be sources of great personal fulfilment and happiness. Yet millions of people are sexually and emotionally dissatisfied. They endure disordered relationships, ranging from plain dull to outright abusive. It doesn't have to be this way – and it shouldn't.

The lack of adequate sex education is a major factor. Young people leave school sexually illiterate. They never get taught the ABC of sex. Schools teach about biology and reproduction, but rarely about sex and relationships. Despite new government guidelines, in reality few pupils receive advice on achieving sexual satisfaction, dealing with emotional problems and rebuffing unwanted sexual advances. Sexual literacy, however, is just as important as literacy in reading and writing. Education is, after all, supposed to prepare young people for later life. Sex and relationships are a very important part of adulthood. Why, then, are they neglected in schools?

The opponents of sex education claim that more information about sex is not the answer. They say kids are already taught enough – or too much! These critics are, however, seriously misinformed. Young people complain that sex education is inadequate and starts late. They want the full facts, but they rarely get them in the classroom; which is why so many teenagers are left with a mixed bag of myths and half-truths picked up from playground gossip and tabloid newspapers.

Teaching about sex is inconsistent, varying widely in different parts of the country. Compared to the Netherlands, the quality ranges from mediocre to very poor and it begins too late – often after young people have become sexually active and have adopted bad habits such as unsafe sex and intercourse without contraception. Lessons tend to be vague and euphemistic. They focus on the biological facts of reproduction – frequently concerning rabbits and guinea pigs, rather than humans. In the better schools there is information about puberty, contraception, pregnancy and safer sex. But this usually lacks sufficient detail and explicitness to be of real practical benefit. There is no glamorization of safer sex to make it an appealing option and no positive promotion of safer alternatives to intercourse, such as fellatio and cunnilingus. Moreover, sex is portrayed overwhelmingly in a negative light, with far too much emphasis on the dangers rather than the pleasures – creating needless fears and anxieties.

Teachers rarely discuss sex itself, let alone how to have a satisfying sex life. They don't promote the idea that sexual rights are human rights and never support the right of young people under the age of consent to make their own choice about when they are ready for sex. Education about emotions and relationships is almost entirely absent.

Homosexuality and bisexuality are likewise often neglected – leaving many lesbian, gay and bisexual pupils feeling isolated and confused and without any specific advice on HIV prevention for same-sex relations. Sexual prejudice, and the teasing and bullying of pupils who don't conform to gender stereotypes, passes unchallenged in many schools. Given the widespread concern about sexual abuse, it is particularly disturbing that most young people never get taught sexual assertiveness and how to deal with unwelcome sexual attention.

These failings point to the need for a radical overhaul of sex education to help resolve the many sexual and emotional problems experienced by young people – problems that often continue into adulthood, causing lifelong personal distress. This essay argues that schools should affirm the value and pleasure of human sexuality, empowering pupils with the knowledge, skills and confidence to make responsible choices that enable them to enjoy a happy, healthy sex life.

MUTUAL RESPECT, CONCERN AND FULFILMENT

Schools cannot be morality-free zones where anything goes. There has to be some kind of moral framework for sex education, otherwise teachers would end up sanctioning all kinds of dangerous, destructive behaviour: coercive and unsafe sex, domineering and violent relationships. A moral framework is not, however, the same as a moralistic one. Both impart ethical values but they differ in one very significant respect: a moralistic framework excludes, whereas a truly moral one is inclusive of different people with diverse backgrounds and lifestyles.

Until very recent times, all sex education was overwhelmingly biased towards promoting heterosexuality, marriage, parenthood and traditional family life. Anything outside this exclusive framework was either ignored or condemned. Knowledge of the full range of consensual sex and love was systematically suppressed. Young people who did not abide by the prevailing sexual orthodoxy – such as gays and bisexuals – were marginalized and often ended up feeling inadequate, guilty, rejected and full of self-loathing.

This old-style monocultural sex moralism is now totally out of sync with our modern multicultural society where there is a great diversity of cultures and communities, lifestyles and love lives. Acknowledging these social changes is, however, no reason to lapse into anarchic moral relativism. Instead, we need a new moral framework for teaching sex education that can encompass diversity while also giving young people guidance on how they are most likely to find erotic and emotional happiness.

This new moral framework involves three very simple principles: mutual respect, consent and fulfilment. In others words, when it comes to lust and love, treat others the way you would like them to treat you. Don't have an egotistical, selfish, me-first attitude. Be thoughtful and caring towards the other person. Never coerce or pressure a partner into doing something they don't want to do. Make sure both of you get physical and psychological enjoyment. That's it! Simple, inclusive and moral – without being moralistic.

These three principles constitute the basis of ethical sex and relationships. Partners should respect each other, act with shared consent and give one another mutual fulfilment. This applies universally, regardless of whether people are heterosexual, homosexual or bisexual; regardless of whether they are married, cohabiting or living apart; regardless of whether they have one partner or many partners; regardless of whether they are into one-night stands or committed relationships; and regardless of whether they have sex for love or sex for pleasure.

The idea that sex within marriage has a monopoly of morality is untrue and offensive, and not just to long-time cohabiting couples. Moral goodness can exist even in casual sex – providing that is what both partners want, they treat each other respect and give one other enjoyment.

Basing sex education on this new moral framework of sexual and emotional mutuality gives young people many options. Instead of straight-jacketing them within an old-style moralism revolving around wedlock, each different individual is free to make his or her own choices, based on his or her own particular feelings, needs and desires. That is how it should be in a pluralistic, multicultural sexual democracy, where the right to be different is a treasured human right.

ALL SEXUALITIES ARE EQUALLY VALID

Within this new moral framework, sexual orientation is no longer an issue, since all sexualities based on mutual consent, respect and fulfilment are equally moral and valid. Until now, however, sex education has been always premised on the doctrine of straight supremacism and sexual apartheid. Heterosexuality has been presented as natural, superior and worthy of exclusive legal privileges, such as the right to marriage. Conversely, if mentioned at all, homosexuality and bisexuality have tended to be seen as inferior – if not downright immoral – and therefore denied full acceptance and validation in the classroom.

The legacy of this heterosexist bias has been the negation of the desires and affections of queer pupils, leaving many with feelings of inadequacy and worthlessness that often contribute to depression, truancy, academic underperformance and even attempted suicide.

Teaching about sex has an ethical responsibility to challenge the prejudice that wrecks the lives of lesbian, gay and bisexual teenagers. While schools should not promote any sexual orientation, they certainly should encourage understanding and acceptance of other people – heterosexual, homosexual and bisexual.

This means presenting the full facts about all three sexual orientations in a straightforward and sympathetic manner. It also involves challenging homophobic attitudes in the school playground and beyond; and providing queer kids with supportive advice and counselling that validates their feelings. The aim must be to help create a caring, compassionate society that values and appreciates everyone, and where young people don't grow up feeling fearful and ashamed of their sexual orientation.

◆ ● ● OPTIONS, NOT PRESCRIPTIONS

In the past, all education was prescriptive. Pupils had to learn 'the facts' and obey 'the rules'. They were taught by rote and had knowledge and morality drummed into them. Every child was expected to share the same values and aspirations. Difference was bad and dangerous. There was no room for questioning or diversity. Teaching has, thankfully, changed. Good schooling nowadays tends to be more critical and reflective and offers a variety of options. It is not about imposing rules and knowledge, but empowering young people to consider the full range of facts and opinions, think for themselves and then choose to make their own informed, responsible choices.

When it comes to sex education that is exactly the way it should be. Different people have different sexual and emotional needs. Our desires and temperaments are not all the same. There is no 'one-size-fits-all' when it comes to sex and love. Some of us are straight, some are queer and some are a bit of both. Sex before marriage is acceptable to most people, but not to everyone. Although monogamy is usually the favoured option, open relationships can also be rewarding. Toe sucking may be the height of sensuality for one person, but a total turnoff for another. There are lovers who prefer to live together and those who like the independence of living apart. Abstinence has its advantages, but so does promiscuity. Marriage is a must for many, but not for cohabiting couples who see love and commitment as more important than legal formality. While oral sex is the ultimate thrill for some, a majority get greatest satisfaction from intercourse – and a few get it from rubber and bondage.

The point is we are all diverse individuals. No two people are the same. What suits you may not suit me. There are diverse ways of finding carnal and emotional fulfilment. That reality should be acknowledged in the classroom. Moreover, the right to sexual difference is just as much a human right as the right to cultural and ethnic difference. That is why teachers have duty to validate the diversity of human sex and relationships that fall within the moral framework of respect, consent, fulfilment and mutuality.

GIVE ALL THE FACTS – TELL THE WHOLE TRUTH

If education is about dispelling ignorance and imparting knowledge, then sex education has an obligation to give all the facts and tell the whole truth about every kind of sex and relationship. This includes sexual practices that some people may find distasteful, such as anal intercourse and sadomasochism, and harmful behaviour like unprotected sex and child abuse. Nothing must be off limits. The purpose of talking frankly about these discomforting issues is not in order to encourage them, but to help pupils cope if they encounter them in later life.

After explaining the full range of sex and relationships, and discussing how they relate to the principles of mutual respect, consent and fulfilment, young people should be trusted to make their own choices. Most will respond to such candour by making sensible, responsible decisions. Those who do not would be reckless anyway, regardless of what they were taught or not taught.

Human sexuality embraces a glorious diversity of feelings, emotions, desires and attractions. We are all unique, with our own unique erotic tastes. People get sexually aroused and fulfilled in a huge variety of different ways. Many of these ways are familiar and accepted. Others, such as anilingus, may seem strange and unpleasant to some people. But difference is the spice of life. One person's sexual nightmare is another person's sexual nirvana. Providing behaviour is consensual, no one is harmed and the enjoyment is reciprocal, schools should adopt a 'live and let live' non-judgemental attitude.

Those who oppose frank sex education protest that young people's innocence must be protected. But it is already too late. Even very young children are aware of sexual issues and erotic exotica. They pick up this information from tabloid newspapers, Hollywood blockbusters, teen magazines, television soaps and classroom banter. Much of this information is, however, half-baked and sensationalist. It can leave kids feeling sexually confused, inadequate, fearful and guilty – which is not conducive to their well being. Honest, explicit sex education has a vital role to play in correcting misinformation and reassuring them with the truth. Young people who know the full facts are more likely to grow up feeling at ease with their sexuality, relate well to their partner and have a contented relationship.

Pupils have a right to know everything about sex, in order to prepare them for desires they may have themselves or may experience with others. Teenagers who are ignorant of cunnilingus, for example, may be shocked when a partner first suggests it. But if they know about oral sex beforehand, they are less likely to be fazed and better able to make an informed judgement about whether it is something they want to do.

To be effective, sex education needs to start at a very early age, beginning gently in the first year of primary school and gradually becoming more detailed and explicit at secondary level. The reason for starting so young is obvious. Children now reach puberty between the ages of eight and 12. Long beforehand, they need to know about the physical changes they will undergo.

The National Survey of Sexual Attitudes and Lifestyles (K. Wellings *et al.*, *Sexual Behaviour in Britain*, 1994) was the world's biggest and most comprehensive sex survey, interviewing over 18,000 people in Britain in 1990. It found that the median age of first sexual experience among 16- to 24-year-olds was 14 for girls and 13 for boys (sexual experience includes everything from touching to kissing, mutual masturbation, oral sex and intercourse). For sexual intercourse, the median age was 17. The research reported that the age of first sex and first intercourse is dropping every decade. A more recent survey, conducted for the Channel 4 television programme *Sex from 8 to 18*, broadcast on 5 July 2000, found that the average age of first intercourse is 15.

If the median age of first sexual experience was 13–14 in 1990 (now probably even lower), and if the average age of first intercourse is now 15, this means a high proportion of young people are sexually active below these ages. That is why sex education has to begin much earlier. It makes no sense to inform young people after they've started having sex. By then it is too late – hence the high incidence of teen pregnancies, abortions and sexually transmitted diseases.

Long before their first experience, young people need to be forearmed with the knowledge, skills and confidence to make wise, responsible sexual decisions – including, of course, the option of not having sex.

Fears that early, explicit sex education will encourage premature and irresponsible sexual experimentation are misplaced. Research by The Alan Guttmacher Institute in the USA (Jones *et al.*, *Teenage Pregnancy in Industrialized Countries*, 1986; *Pregnancy, Contraception and Family Planning Services in Industrialized Countries*, 1989) found that the lowest rates of teenage pregnancies and abortions are found in countries with the most liberal sexual attitudes, the frankest sex lessons in schools and the most widely available family planning services.

SEX IS GOOD FOR YOU

Sex education is mostly anti-sex. It focuses on the potential negative consequences, such as unwanted pregnancies and HIV infection. There are endless warnings about the risks and pitfalls. Moralism is rife: don't do this, don't do that. The nasty consequences of the more sensational sexual diseases get plenty of coverage. Impotence! Infertility! Insanity! This erotophobic bias sends out the message that sex is bad and dangerous. It fuels the sex psychosis that makes young people fearful and anxious about a human activity that ought to be a source of great pleasure and joy.

Sex lessons should tell the truth: sex is good for us. It is natural, wholesome, fun and healthy. Good sex can have a very positive, beneficial effect on our mental and physical well-being; lifting our spirits and creating new-found energy and optimism. The exhilarating rush and release of a powerful orgasm can have profound psychic reverberations, creating feelings of elation, cleansing, inner peace and sublime contentment. It is no accident that surveys of human happiness have often found a high correlation between being happy and being sexually fulfilled. The two tend to go together.

Research by Dr Merryn Gott of Sheffield University ('Long Live Loving', *Daily Mail*, 10 September 2001) found that having an enjoyable sex life boosts a person's self-esteem, confidence and sense of well-being. It also discovered that good sex helps sustain a good relationship; easing tensions and strengthening feelings of togetherness and commitment. Young people have a right to know that while sex is not essential for health and happiness (some mystics get by without it), most people find that regular, quality sex enhances their lives.

OVERCOMING GUILT AND SHAME

Sex is not dirty. The naked human body is not obscene. Homosexuality is not immoral. Why, then, do schools do so little to challenge the Victorian-style sexphobia that still wrecks the lives of so many people?

Lots of adults feel ill at ease undressing and being naked in front of their partner. Some can only have sex in the dark, in a bed and in the conventional way. Many are so fearful of sexual pleasure that they barely make a sound when they climax. Some cannot cope with anything other than quick, furtive liaisons. Others suffer from post-sex guilt and depression. Plenty feel anxious about same-sex desires.

Sexual shame causes immense human misery: not just frustrated, unhappy sex lives, but actual psychological and physical ill health. Phobias, neuroses, panic attacks and eating disorders can sometimes originate from guilt about sex. Ignoring or tolerating the internalized puritanism that causes sexual and emotional dysfunction is incompatible with the ethos of a responsible education system, which is to care for the present and future welfare of children.

There is, therefore, a moral obligation on schools to challenge sex-shame pathology. Youngsters should be encouraged to feel relaxed and comfortable with their bodies and sexuality. The best way to achieve this is by talking openly and frankly about any and every sexual issue that concerns them. Sexual pleasure ought to be normalized and legitimated by treating it like any other form of pleasure: it is something to enjoy and feel good about.

There is another very important reason why teachers should challenge anxieties about sex. Sexual shame helps sustain child abuse. Adults who sexually exploit youngsters often get away with it because the victims feel embarrassed or guilty about sex and are therefore reluctant to complain. This reluctance is reinforced by strait-laced cultural attitudes, which tend still to regard sex as something sordid that should be kept hidden and private. These attitudes are a godsend to abusers, who depend on guilt and secrecy to carry out their molestation undetected.

To combat the sexual shame that inhibits the exposure of abusers, sex education lessons need to encourage young people to have more open and positive attitudes towards sexual matters. Teenagers who feel at ease talking about sex are more likely to disclose abuse.

◈● ●
● ●
● ● ◈ **HOW TO HAVE GOOD, SAFE SEX**

Most pupils leave school with little idea of how to have good sex. They sometimes can't please themselves, let alone their partners. The end result is bad sex and mutual dissatisfaction.

Senior-level sex education should include advice on how to achieve mutually fulfilling, high-quality sex – the emotional and erotic value of foreplay, the multitude of erogenous zones and how to excite them and the importance of deep breathing and strong, rhythmic muscle contractions to the achievement of good orgasms.

Men and women understand very little about each other's bodies and how they work sexually. This ignorance results in frequent disappointment, especially for women. Boys need to be taught that intercourse is not the be-all-and-end-all of sex. Finger stimulation of the clitoris can produce stronger orgasms than penile penetration. There should also be frank advice on remedies for sexual problems such as impotence, frigidity, erotic phobias, inability to achieve orgasm and premature ejaculation.

When it comes to good sex, many people see safer sex as second best. It is, therefore, important that teachers promote safer sex as a different, not inferior, way of achieving sexual enjoyment.

Successful HIV prevention campaigns have shown that the most effective way to encourage the adoption of safer sex is by using sexy images that make playing safe look desirable and glamorous. Giving risk reduction sex appeal gets results. Preaching at young people doesn't.

Schools should learn from this experience. Instead of presenting safer sex exclusively as a duty and responsibility, teachers should also promote it as an attractive, sexy alternative. Clinical, medical explanations of non-risky behaviour need to be ditched in favour of sexually explicit 'how to' guides that eroticize condom use and non-penetrative sex as fun and fulfilling. This means presenting arousing images that create a mental connection between getting turned on and playing safe.

To help combat the view that condoms are a bore and a sacrifice, lessons should highlight their positive advantages: they enable men to keep going stronger and longer. Many guys suffer from premature ejaculation. By reducing sensitivity, a condom can prolong staying power and intensify orgasm, giving enhanced pleasure to both partners.

Teachers need to challenge the idea that sex equals intercourse. That is what most people think. Everything else tends to be dismissed as kid's stuff and mere foreplay. Screwing is the 'real thing'. This is a very narrow, limiting view of sex, which the education system does nothing to debunk.

If schools are serious about cutting the incidence of teenage pregnancies, abortions and HIV infections, they should actively encourage safer, healthier alternatives to intercourse. Oral sex and mutual masturbation carry no risk of conception and a low risk of HIV. Promoting these alternatives, therefore, makes good sense.

The best way to persuade teenagers to adopt oral sex and mutual masturbation is by making them look and sound sexy and by emphasizing their advantages over intercourse: no worries about unwanted conceptions, no need to use the pill or condoms and no dependence on a man's ability to get and stay erect.

Good sex tends to involve emotional input. Yet emotional issues are almost entirely ignored in the classroom. If they were discussed more, lots of teenagers might be spared great distress. Schools advise students that sex within a relationship is best but, astonishingly, they never teach them how to sustain a good relationship: the importance of honesty, negotiation, compatibility, trust, reciprocity, give and take and spontaneity. There is no practical advice on how to deal with disagreements and difficulties. What do you do if your boyfriend refuses to use a condom? What is the best way to respond when a partner takes you for granted? Breaking up can be a very traumatic experience, yet pupils get no guidance on how to cope with splitting up and how to deal with the pain of rejection.

SEXUAL RIGHTS ARE HUMAN RIGHTS

The right to love a person of either sex, to engage in any mutually consensual sexual act, and to enjoy a happy, healthy sex life is a fundamental human right. This right to sexual self-determination should be promoted in every school, to create a culture of sexual rights where every young person understands and asserts their right to determine what they, and others, do with their body. This ethos of 'it's my body, I'm in charge' is the best possible protection against people who try to manipulate and pressure youngsters into having sex.

The Dutch have proved the positive benefits of actively promoting the right of young people to make their own decisions about when they are ready for a sexual relationship. Far from being a licence for reckless sex, this freedom is generally exercised with care and wisdom. Teenagers in the Netherlands are more likely than their British counterparts to resist peer pressure to experiment sexually at an early age. On average, they have their first sexual intercourse when they are older and they have rates of teenage pregnancies and abortions seven times lower than those of the UK.

One of the most important sexual human rights is the right not be abused. For a society that professes such concern about sexual abuse, it is curious the way the issue is rarely, if ever, mentioned in the classroom. When it is raised, kids are mostly warned about 'stranger danger', which is simplistic and inadequate. Most abuse is perpetrated by carers and family members. It usually involves seduction, not abduction. Coercion and violence are rare. Psychological pressure and manipulation is common. Yet few pupils receive assertiveness training on how to say no to sex pests or advice on what to do if a parent, teacher or care worker is molesting them. Telling kids to phone Childline is not enough. They need to be taught the ability and assuredness to reject and report unwelcome sexual attention.

Bizarrely, the law places no obligation on schools to provide young people with the knowledge, skills and confidence that would help them stand up to abusers. Education in abuse issues should be key component of sex education. As the Dutch have long realized, the best protection against sexual abuse is earlier, better quality sex education. Young people need to be educated and empowered to stick up for their sexual rights, which include both the right to say 'yes' to sex and the right to say 'no'. Teenagers who are knowledgeable and confident about sexual matters – and who are aware that they have the right to control their own body – are much more likely to reject undesired sexual overtures and, if abuse occurs, to speak out.

◈●●
 ●　●
 ●●◈ CONCLUSION

These ideas for the reform of sex education are plain common sense, which is why they are commonplace in many north European schools. The results speak for themselves: wiser, more responsible sexual behaviour.

Keeping young people in a state of sexual ignorance, disempowerment, ineptitude and dissatisfaction is a form of child abuse. It disfigures lives, creating untold erotic and emotional misery. The right to sexual health and happiness is a fundamental human right. It is time the school system prioritized sexual literacy, alongside literacy in words and numbers, to ensure that future generations live erotically and emotionally fulfilled lives in a mature, enlightened sexual democracy.

AFTERWORD
Ellie Lee and Tiffany Jenkins

The essays in this collection suggest that disagreements about what schools should teach children in sex education centre on two main issues: the role of sex education in alleviating 'sexual health' problems, and its role in preparing young people for adult life. Differences of opinion on these issues can be summarized as follows.

SEX EDUCATION AND SEXUAL HEALTH PROBLEMS

SEX EDUCATION IS VITAL TO REDUCE THE INCIDENCE OF POOR SEXUAL HEALTH

Those who advocate the provision of sex education in schools argue that 'sexual health' problems are a major cause for concern. They are convinced that a compelling argument for the provision of sex education is that it can help reduce such problems, in particular, rates of teenage pregnancy and of sexually transmitted infections (STIs).

Proponents of this argument tend to believe, however, that it is unrealistic to deal with these problems simply by discouraging young people from having sex at all. That it is possible to generate a society where the risk of sexual health problems is reduced through young people abstaining from sex until marriage is an untenable proposition. Rather, it is argued, society must accept that young people do have sex in their teenage years and that sex education in schools plays an absolutely central role in improving the sexual health of young people.

In this framework, there is a clear relationship between the knowledge young people receive at school and their sexual practices. The more young people are taught about sex, the less they will engage in sexual practices that put their health at risk. Equipping young people with knowledge about sex is therefore the first step in reducing the likelihood that they will take risks. Sex education can also bring about a situation where young people delay having sex, through empowering them to combat 'peer pressure' and can help ensure that when they do, they practice 'safer sex' – by using contraception.

Among those who agree that sex education plays a crucial role in combating sexual health problems are those who contend that, too often, sex education is unhelpfully negative about sex. Sex, they argue, is often presented as a source of disease and emotional problems, rather than a source of pleasure and enjoyment. Such 'sex negativity' does young people a disservice in that it fails to communicate the positive role that sex plays in people's lives. From this perspective, good sex education would promote safer sex, but would do so in such a way that encourages sexual experimentation and avoids stigmatizing sex.

SEX EDUCATION MAKES SEXUAL HEALTH PROBLEMS WORSE

A stronger criticism of sex education is that it encourages promiscuous behaviour. This argument is often perceived to be the counterpoint to that just summarized, but in fact it begins from the same starting point – that rates of teenage pregnancy and of STIs are major social problems. This is where agreement ends however. To date, it is argued, sex education has not only manifestly failed to tackle poor sexual health among the young, but has encouraged its emergence. Through condoning sex outside marriage and refusing to present stable heterosexual unions as the morally appropriate environment in which to raise children, it has encouraged promiscuity and the health problems associated with it. From this perspective sex education can only reduce rates of teenage pregnancy and STIs if it acts as a vector for morally correct messages about the importance of family life and the sanctity of marriage.

THE PROBLEM OF SEXUAL HEALTH – A MATTER OF VALUES, NOT FACTS

A third approach takes a different starting point from either of the two above, in that it questions the notion that sexual health problems are as serious as is often suggested. This approach contends that those who advocate sex education on the grounds that teenage pregnancy and sexually transmitted infections are major social problems often exaggerate the risks young people face and fail to base their arguments on the facts of the matter. In the terms of this argument, while the case for sex education on the grounds of improving sexual health may sound factual, scientific and morally neutral, it is in fact highly value laden. In highlighting the alleged health risks of sex, such sex education deems certain forms of sexual behaviour 'morally responsible' (for example, non-penetrative sex) and stigmatizes others as problematic (for example, sex without contraception). The logic of this case is that while young people may need improved access to contraception and need to know how to avoid contracting or treat STIs, they do not need to be taught in school that sex is a risky business.

◆ ● ●
● ● **THE ROLE OF SEX EDUCATION IN EQUIPPING**
● ● ◆ **YOUNG PEOPLE FOR ADULT LIFE**

SEX AND RELATIONSHIPS EDUCATION IS ESSENTIAL IN PROVIDING A
VALUES FRAMEWORK FOR YOUNG PEOPLE

Many who argue in support of sex and relationships education contend
it plays an essential part in the process of educating young people, by
providing them with a 'values framework'. Sex and relationships
education, they suggest, has a vital role to play, together with PHSE
and citizenship education, in encouraging young people to adopt a set
of values that can guide them in their interaction with others.

The use of the term 'values' is important in this argument. A 'values
framework' is above all 'non-judgemental'. It seeks to avoid making
overt judgements – for example, that it is only possible to bring up
children well where parents are married or that heterosexuality is
'normal' and homosexuality 'abnormal'. And it is careful not to make
the case that sexual activity on the part of teenagers is a problem –
it fully accepts that teenagers often have sex.

However, proponents of this 'values framework' argue this does not
mean it is value free. Rather, emphasis is placed on acquiring
attitudes and values that can enable young people to conduct their
relationships with others in an appropriate way. These include
'respect for others', 'respect for difference' (for example in relation
to ethnicity, sexual orientation or disability), the importance of 'love
and care' and of 'self-esteem'.

Some who believe that sex education should be about 'values' rather
than moralism contend that sex education has to be radically
transformed before it achieves this goal. While encouraging young

people to respect others and show concern for them is the framework that should guide sex and relationships education in schools, too often this is not the case. Instead, such critics argue, homosexuality, sex for pleasure (for example, in 'one-night stands') or single parenthood are still often treated as undesirable and deemed outside the bounds of a 'values framework'.

YOUNG PEOPLE NEED MORALS, NOT VALUES

Others, while agreeing that young people do need to be provided with a framework to guide their interaction with others, contend that 'morality', in its traditional sense, should be championed. In the terms of this argument, those who advocate 'values' are merely accommodating to and accepting low standards of behaviour, with disastrous consequences. Once the notion is abandoned that marriage, family life and heterosexuality are normal and are the best ways to live life and bring up children, significant social disintegration will inevitably occur. As society becomes de-moralized, young people become unable to make judgements about what is right and wrong and once this happens, social ills associated with the decline of marriage and a loss of respect for the family multiply. If children are to be taught about relationships in schools the notion that marriage, fidelity and family life are superior to other ways of living, must be the cornerstone of such education.

WHO NEEDS SEX EDUCATION?

The idea that 'morals' and 'values' exist in opposition to one another is called into question by a third outlook. Those arguing from this standpoint contend first, that apparently 'non-judgemental' values can be just as prescriptive and controlling as the morals they are supposed to replace. For example, the argument that differences must be respected, can lead to the stigmatization of playground banter (as an alleged manifestation of 'sexism' or 'racism'), the problematization of what is little more than immaturity which adolescents will grow out of anyway and thus will increase the supervision of young people's lives.

Underpinning this criticism of both 'morals' and 'values' is a rejection of the notion that young people need to be taught how to behave properly through sex education in schools. In contrast, proponents of this argument contend, young people can and will be socialized without specific lessons about relationships in schools and, indeed, are more likely to learn how to be independent, and how to negotiate relationships with others effectively, if their space is not colonized by adults. In the terms of this case, whether sex education purports to control or 'empower' young people is irrelevant. In either case, it does more harm than good.

A clear sense emerges from this collection of essays that disagreements continue to exist about what schools should teach children about sex. What sex education sets out to achieve and whether it can achieve its stated goals remain issues for debate. Arguably, the implication for policy makers is that until there is firm evidence for the efficacy of sex education programmes, in relation to their stated goals, it is worth erring on the side of caution, lest schools are set the task of delivering outcomes they are unable to achieve.

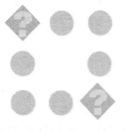

DEBATING MATTERS

Institute of Ideas
Expanding the Boundaries of Public Debate

If you have found this book interesting, and agree that 'debating matters', you can find out more about the Institute of Ideas and our programme of live conferences and debates by visiting our website **www.instituteofideas.com**.
Alternatively you can email **info@instituteofideas.com**
or call 020 7269 9220 to receive a full programme of events and information about joining the Institute of Ideas.

Other titles available in this series:

DEBATING MATTERS

Institute of Ideas
Expanding the Boundaries of Public Debate

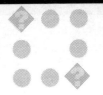

SCIENCE:

CAN WE TRUST THE EXPERTS?

Controversies surrounding a plethora of issues, from the MMR vaccine to mobile phones, from BSE to genetically-modified foods, have led many to ask how the public's faith in government advice can be restored. At the heart of the matter is the role of the expert and the question of whose opinion to trust.

In this book, prominent participants in the debate tell us their views:

- Bill Durodié, who researches risk and precaution at New College, Oxford University
- Dr Ian Gibson MP, Chairman of the Parliamentary Office of Science and Technology
- Dr Sue Mayer, Executive Director of Genewatch UK
- Dr Doug Parr, Chief Scientist for Greenpeace UK.

DESIGNER BABIES:

WHERE SHOULD WE DRAW THE LINE?

Science fiction has been preoccupied with technologies to control the characteristics of our children since the publication of Aldous Huxley's *Brave New World*. Current arguments about 'designer babies' almost always demand that lines should be drawn and regulations tightened. But where should regulation stop and patient choice in the use of reproductive technology begin?

The following contributors set out their arguments:

- Juliet Tizzard, advocate for advances in reproductive medicine
- Professor John Harris, ethicist
- Veronica English and Ann Sommerville of the British Medical Association
- Josephine Quintavalle, pro-life spokesperson
- Agnes Fletcher, disability rights campaigner.